Allergy
Allergy

Chris Corrigan

Reader and Consultant
Department of Asthma, Allergy and Respiratory Science
Guy's, King's & St Thomas' School of Medicine
London, UK

Sabina Rak

Professor of Allergology
Asthma and Allergy Research Group
Department of Respiratory Medicine and Allergy
Sahlgrenska University Hospital
Göteborg, Sweden

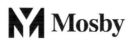 Mosby

MOSBY
An imprint of Elsevier Limited.

© 2004 Elsevier Limited.

The
Publisher's
policy is to use
**paper manufactured
from sustainable forests**

M Mosby is a registered trademark of Elsevier Limited.

ISBN 0-7234-3377-1

Cataloguing in Publication Data
Catalogue records for this book are available from the US Library of Congress
and the British Library.

Note
Medical knowledge is constantly changing. As new information becomes
available, changes in treatment, procedures, equipment and the use of drugs
become necessary. The editors/authors/contributors and the publishers have
taken care to ensure that the information given in this text is accurate and up
to date. However, readers are strongly advised to confirm that the information, especially with regard to drug usage, complies with the latest legislation
and standards of practice.

Printed in China.

Acknowledgements

I acknowledge gratefully the patience and resilience of my secretary Pamela Robertin. Thanks Pam.
I acknowledge the help of Anne Rhiannon, Jonathan and Philip – just for being there.

Chris Corrigan

I acknowledge the love and companionship of my husband David.

Sabina Rak

Contents

Abbreviations

ACE	angiotensin converting enzyme
ARIA	WHO Initiative on Allergic Rhinitis and its Impact on Asthma
BTS	British Thoracic Society
ESR	erythrocyte sedimentation rate
FEV	forced expiratory volume
IEI	idiopathic environmental intolerance
NSAIDS	non-steroidal anti-inflammatory drugs
PEF	peak expiratory flow
RAST	radioallergosorbent test
RCP	Royal College of Physicians
SIGN	Scottish Intercollegiate Guidelines Network

Definition, pathogenesis and epidemiology

What is allergy?

Allergy is one of a group of diseases arising from inappropriate over-reaction of the immune system to antigens. These "hypersensitivity" responses are exaggerated and cause illness. Allergic reactions, classified as Type I or "immediate" hypersensitivity because of their rapid onset, arise from an inappropriate production in some individuals of IgE antibody to antigens ("allergens") encountered at the mucosal surfaces of the skin, conjunctiva, respiratory and gastrointestinal tracts. Patients with a propensity to produce such IgE are termed "atopic".

Table 1 lists diseases that are IgE-mediated and those that are not but sometimes fall in the realm of referral of the allergist. Diseases in the last three categories of this table are best managed by other specialists. The principal role of the allergist when faced with diseases in the second category (Table 1) is to rule out a contribution of allergy to the disease. For diseases in the third and fifth categories, the allergist may play some role in the multidisciplinary approach that is often necessary.

The burden of allergic disease

The huge burden of allergic disease has been estimated in the recent report of a working party of the Royal College of Physicians (RCP).[1] In any one year, over 20% of the population (12 million people) have an active allergic disease needing management, and this number continues to grow. Allergic diseases may have a profound effect on quality of life, and are one of the leading causes of time spent off school or work. Many allergic disorders co-exist in the same patient, emphasizing the disadvantage of having these patients managed by a single-organ specialist. Allergy care

Table 1. Diseases appropriately or inappropriately referred to an allergist

Classical IgE-mediated (atopic) disease[*]
- Atopic rhinitis (includes hayfever)
- Atopic asthma
- Immediate allergic reactions to foods
- Anaphylactic reactions
- Urticaria/angioedema
- Atopic dermatitis (eczema)
- Drug allergy
- Insect venom allergy
- Latex allergy

Non-IgE-mediated disorders[*]
- Non-atopic rhinitis
- Non-atopic asthma
- Food intolerance
- Idiopathic and physical urticaria
- Non-atopic eczema
- Non-immediate drug reactions

Conditions sometimes attributable to non-immunological reactions to external agents[†]
- Irritable bowel syndrome
- Migraine

Other hypersensitivity syndromes not mediated by IgE[†]
- Contact dermatitis
- Extrinsic allergic alveolitis
- Coeliac disease (gluten-induced enteropathy)

Conditions sometimes incorrectly attributed to allergy[†]
- Chronic fatigue syndrome
- Some psychological disturbances and somatization disorders
- Hyperventilation

[*]Within the domain of the allergist.
[†]Not within the domain of the allergist.

in the community alone costs the NHS an estimated £900 million every year, mostly from prescribed treatments in primary care (10% of the GP's prescribing budget). Currently, 6% of all GP consultations are for allergic disease.

The RCP report has highlighted the appalling lack of resources in hospitals and the community for the management of patients with allergic disease. Pressure must be brought to bear on hospital trusts, primary care trusts and strategic planners to ensure that this situation is remedied.

Sources of outdoor inhaled allergens

The National Pollen Monitoring Network in the UK, based at Worcester, provides information on the timing of pollen and spore seasons (see http://pollenuk.worc.ac.uk). A list of all the allergens contained in pollens, spores and dander may be found at www.allergen.org.

Many allergenic types of pollen are found in the UK. Grass pollen allergy is by far the most important, and is seen in 95% of hayfever sufferers. The main flowering season is from late May until the beginning of August. The second most important pollen is birch pollen (Figure 1), to which 25% of hayfever sufferers are allergic. Birch trees "flower" during April and May. Their pollen cross-reacts with the pollen of other members of the birch family, including alder and hazel, which flower earlier, and hornbeam, which flowers later. The main weed allergenic pollens in the UK include nettle, plantain, dock and goosefoot. The peak pollen season for weeds is in late summer and early autumn. Fungal spores, which may cause allergy, are ubiquitous and local concentrations vary with season, vegetation, land use and weather. The most

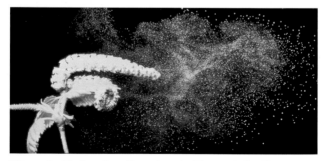

Figure 1. Birch pollen. Reproduced with permission from Corrigan C, Klimek L, Hörmann K. *Rhinitis: Illustrated Differential Diagnosis*. London: Mosby. 2001.

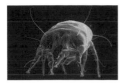

Figure 2. House dust mite. Reproduced with permission from Mac Cochrane G, Jackson WF, Rees PJ. *Asthma: Current Perspectives*. London: Mosby-Wolfe1996.

important are *Cladosporium, Alternaria, Aspergillus* and *Penicillium*. Pollen concentrations are generally higher inland and in the countryside. Local weather conditions such as thunderstorms[2] and pollution[3] can result in increased allergen release.

Sources of indoor inhaled allergens

One leading source of indoor allergens in all houses is the house dust mite (Figure 2). These small creatures live in mattresses, pillows and cushions, and in general are found wherever dust accumulates. Gut enzymes and other proteins present in their faeces are powerful allergens. They thrive in poorly ventilated, warm and humid atmospheres. They are responsible for allergic exacerbation of asthma, rhinitis and eczema throughout the year.

Domestic pets are the second most important source of indoor allergens in the UK. Allergic reactions to furred domestic pets and laboratory animals such as rats and mice occur frequently. Allergenic proteins from the gut, urine or skin of these animals become trapped in airborne dander. Many such allergens are transported out of homes, for example stuck to clothing. The only way to reduce exposure to pets at home is not to have one,[4] although even after removal of the pet it may take many months for the allergen reservoir to diminish.

Fungal and other spores may be a significant source of allergens in the home, especially where there are damp conditions. *Aspergillus* and *Penicillium* are chief culprits.

Pathogenesis and treatment of allergic diseases

Cellular mechanisms

All reactions against foreign proteins, including allergens, are initiated by T lymphocytes. CD4 T cells influence inflammatory reactions by secreting a range of proteins called cytokines, which regulate infiltration and activation of particular granulocytes into the tissues, and the amount and type of antibodies made by B lymphocytes (which are responsible for making all antibodies, including IgE).

CD4 T cells have been further subdivided into Th1, Th2 and Th0, according to the principal cytokines that they produce, which in turn reflects their pro-inflammatory properties. Th2 T cells produce the cytokines IL-4, IL-5 and IL-13, which play a critical role in the regulation of allergic inflammation.[5,6] A scheme of the pathogenesis of allergic inflammation is shown in Figure 3. Allergen-activated Th2 T cells release cytokines, such as IL-5, which attract and activate eosinophils (Eo), which release toxic granule proteins and leukotrienes, causing tissue damage and chronic symptoms depending on the target organ (bronchial obstruction and hyperreactivity, nasal blockage, chronic eczema).[7] Allergen-specific B lymphocytes also interact with allergen-specific Th2 T cells and are thus stimulated to produce allergen-specific antibodies. Under the influence of the Th2 cytokines IL-4 and IL-13, these antibodies are "switched" to the IgE isotype: this is the basis of the inappropriate production of allergen-specific IgE antibody that defines atopy. IgE is able to coat mast cells (MC) by binding to their high-affinity IgE receptors, thus "priming" the cells to degranulate acutely on further encounter with allergens, which cross-link surface-bound IgE. Upon degranulation, mast cells release a distinct array of pro-inflammatory mediators including histamine,

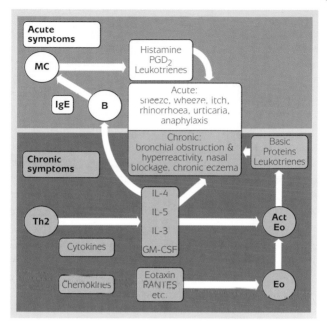

Figure 3. Schematic diagram of the pathogenesis of allergic inflammation (see text for further explanation).

leukotrienes, prostaglandins and proteases. These mediators are responsible for acute symptoms of allergic disease (acute wheeze and sneeze, rhinorrhoea, itch, urticaria, acute exacerbation of eczema and anaphylaxis).

Pharmacological therapy

Drugs which inhibit T cell function, particularly corticosteroids, reduce local cytokine production, eosinophil infiltration and chronic symptoms. This is why topical corticosteroids are such effective prophylactic agents, although they have little direct inhibitory affect on mast cell degranulation and so do not relieve acute symptoms immediately. Furthermore, corticosteroids do little to reduce IgE production by B cells once this is established, and so cannot be used to "treat" inappropriate

IgE responses. Conversely, drugs which inhibit the effects of mast cell products, particularly antihistamines, relieve acute symptoms without much affecting the underlying inflammation, and so are inappropriate as prophylactic therapy. Since leukotrienes are released by both mast cells and eosinophils, leukotriene antagonists might be expected to inhibit both the acute and chronic manifestations of allergic disease, although those currently available for therapeutic use in the UK (montelukast, zafirlukast) block only the effects of eosinophil-derived leukotrienes.

A subset of smaller protein messengers called chemokines also play an important role in recruitment of cells to sites of allergic inflammation.[9] These mediators have a special function of chemically attracting particular cells according to the chemokine receptors they express, and also promoting their migration out of the capillary circulation into tissue (diapedesis).

It should be noted that a proportion of so called "non-atopic" patients with asthma, eczema and rhinitis do not make detectable IgE, at least in the circulation, against allergens. Consequently, they do not have acute exacerbation of disease following allergen exposure. In all other respects, however, they have evidence of Th2 T cell activation, Th2 cytokine production and eosinophil infiltration of the target organs, and respond to corticosteroid therapy.

Unanswered questions in allergy

Despite the tidy-looking scenario above, which is based on decades of research, there are many more fundamental questions pertaining to the pathogenesis of allergic disease which remain to be addressed. Some of these include:

- Why, upon equivalent exposure to inhaled or ingested allergens, do only some individuals make allergen-specific IgE?
- Why do many subjects who develop allergen-specific IgE not develop allergic diseases?
- Why do allergic diseases develop within an individual in some target organs but not others?
- Why do some allergic diseases regress clinically while the IgE response persists?
- Why do individuals differ so widely in their clinical sensitivity to particular allergens?
- Why is the pattern of responses to different allergens variable and not heritable?

These observations remain unexplained, but do emphasise the fact that the presence of allergen-specific IgE, while required for the diagnosis of allergy, is not predictive of the presence or severity of clinical symptoms. They also imply that there may be intrinsic differences in the structure or physiology of target organs which allow disease to develop in some individuals but not in others. There are very few indications as to where this variability, if it does indeed exist, might lie.

Diagnostic tests for allergy

Specific IgE antibody against various allergens can be demonstrated by a skin prick test or measuring specific IgE in the serum.

Skin prick tests are sensitive, cheap and easy to perform once staff are trained. Glycerol suspensions of allergens are placed onto the skin and pricked gently into the epidermis with a sterile metal lancet (Figure 4). The position of each allergen is marked with a biro. Negative (diluent) controls (since some patients with dermographism react to any skin insult with a wheal) and positive (histamine) controls (since the test is dimished and therefore invalidated if patients are taking oral antihistamines, oral steroids or using topical steroid creams) are essential. If the subject is sensitized to a particular allergen, local mast cell degranulation with histamine release produces a wheal, the size of which (orthogonal diameters) is measured and recorded at 15 minutes (Figure 5). A wide variety of allergen extracts for skin prick testing is available from various commercial sources. These tests can be safely performed by trained personnel in the community.

While many allergen extracts are stable, those from fruits and vegetables may decay rapidly on storage, making skin prick tests unreliable. In such cases, it is better to perform a "prick-prick" test where the lancet is used to prick the fruit/vegetable in question and then the patient. This

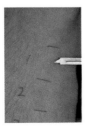

Figure 4. Skin prick testing with a lancet. Reproduced with permission from Corrigan C, Klimek L, Hörmann K. *Rhinitis: Illustrated Differential Diagnosis*. London: Mosby. 2001.

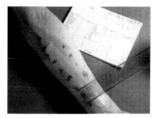

Figure 5. Reading the skin prick test result. Reproduced with permission from Corrigan C, Klimek L, Hörmann K. *Rhinitis: Illustrated Differential Diagnosis*. London: Mosby. 2001.

principle may also be extended to other suspect articles such as rubber gloves (see relevant sections).

The measurement of allergen-specific IgE in serum is now widely available and sophisticated. Radioallergosorbent tests (RAST) have now been replaced with ELISA tests, which are becoming increasingly quantitative. RAST may be performed where skin prick tests are unavailable or impracticable, or in very highly sensitized patients in whom a possible anaphylactic reaction to the skin prick test is considered a possibility (exceedingly rare). Nevertheless, RAST are less sensitive and much more expensive than skin prick tests, and do not furnish an immediate result.

All of these tests are of limited use without a detailed clinical history, since the presence of allergen-specific IgE does not predict the presence, or severity, of clinical allergic reactions. They may confirm the involvement of IgE-mediated reactions already suspected from the history, but cannot be used prospectively to "predict" allergic reactions. Having said this, quantitative RAST have some value in predicting the likelihood of remission of some allergic diseases such as peanut allergy (see chapter on Food Allergy).

Special challenge tests may be need to make the diagnosis of allergy, for example to foods and drugs (see relevant sections), often where there are no validated skin prick tests, the mechanism does not involve IgE, or when it is necessary to demonstrate the lack of reactivity to a patient. Allergen inhalation tests can confirm suspected causes of occupational asthma. These tests are day-case procedures in specialist allergy units with facilities and expertise for treating anaphylaxis.

Epidemiology and primary prevention of allergy

Overt manifestations of atopy typically develop in childhood, often starting with cow's milk allergy and atopic dermatitis, which usually occur within the first year of life but frequently resolve in later life. The later progression of disease to chronic atopic dermatitis, rhinoconjunctivitis and asthma has been termed the "atopic march".[10,11] While this tidy scenario suggests a process of progression of early immunological sensitization towards clinical disease, it should be remembered that allergic diseases may also appear at any time in life, while IgE-mediated diseases may remit at least clinically.

Numerous epidemiological and cohort studies have emphasised that allergic disease represents a major and increasing health problem in many industrialized countries, and that IgE-mediated diseases result from a complex interaction of genetic predisposition (see later) and environmental exposure.[12-14] The rapid increase in prevalence over the last 20 years cannot be accounted for by genetic shift within the population. Rather, changes in living conditions and/or environmental factors are much more likely to have contributed to this increase. The corollary is that such factors can potentially be identified and reversed.

The observation that allergic disease is an epidemic in developed, Westernized society has led to the emergence of the *hygiene hypothesis*, which proposes that the absence or reduction of microbial factors stimulating the immune system, particularly early in life through the use of sterilized foodstuffs, antibiotics, vaccination and the like has facilitated the development of allergen-driven immune reactions, resulting ultimately in allergic disease.[15] This hypothesis is supported by epidemiological findings showing a reduced risk of developing allergic diseases later in life in children with increasing numbers of siblings,[16] early attendance at day-care facilities,[17] frequent infections in the first year of life[18] and frequent orofaecal viral infections[19] (considered a general reflection of "poor hygiene"). Moreover, a protective effect on the development of allergic diseases has been noted in children spending the first years of their life on farms,[20] where it has been postulated that they are exposed to endotoxin, present in the cell walls of numerous human and animal bacteria and their excreta.[21] The hypothesis underlying all these observations is that viral and bacterial infections, as well as endotoxin exposure, may "push" T cell responses away from Th2 towards Th1, although this extension of the hygiene hypothesis remains controversial and other, perhaps more significant, environmental factors may come to light in the future.

Building on this hypothesis, it has been shown in animal models of allergic disease that immune stimulators or modifying agents (*immune response modifiers*) such as heat killed bacteria[22] or CpG oligonucleotides[23] may modify immune responses away from Th2 towards Th1 during primary exposure to allergens, but it will be a long time before the safety and efficacy of these procedures justify their use in newborn children.

It is unlikely that allergen avoidance has any practical role to play in primary allergy prevention. Allergen sensitization may occur *in utero* from maternal transmission of allergens.[24] After birth, avoidance of most allergens is impossible or of limited, probably transient efficacy[25] and, even if it reduces the likelihood of being sensitized in early childhood, it does not necessarily obviate the possibility later in life.

Identification of "at-risk" children

Primary prevention strategies might best be directed at "at-risk" children. Family history remains the best predictor of risk: a child with one atopic parent has a 40–60% risk of developing atopy. With both parents atopic, this risk rises to 60–80%, whereas with neither parent atopic it is only 5%. Intensive activity is currently in progress to define this genetic risk element of atopy. There are two basic approaches. The "candidate gene" approach relies on the identification of slight variations, or polymorphisms in the DNA sequence of genes in different individuals which may affect the expression or function of their corresponding protein products. The frequency of particular polymorphisms in "candidate genes" (that is, those thought to encode proteins such as cytokines relevant to allergic inflammation) is compared in allergic and non-allergic individuals.[26] Such studies have linked numerous polymorphisms in the q31-33 region of chromosome 5, which contains several Th2 cytokine genes, and many other polymorphisms elsewhere with the allergic phenotype, although the precise implications of these findings in pathogenetic terms are often unknown. The second approach, "gene screening", follows the inheritance of markers or "satellites" on particular chromosomes with the inheritance of atopy in the offspring in family studies. Statistical techniques allow the pinpointing of specific areas of chromosomes, the inheritance of which predisposes to allergic disease. The advantage of this technique is that it does not involve *a priori* assumptions about which genes may be important. The disadvantage is that genes within suspect regions of chromosomes may be difficult to pinpoint precisely. One recent success with this technique has been the identification of the ADAM 33 gene,[27] which encodes a proteinase secreted by normal fibroblast and smooth muscle cells within the lung, which may be involved in normal tissue remodelling. This finding is of particular interest, since it provides the first pointer that allergic disease may reflect inherited abnormalities in target organs rather than immunological processes (see discussion above).

Despite these advances and intensive research, it will likely be a long time before gene screening can be used accurately to predict the likelihood of any individual developing atopy, let alone particular atopic diseases.

Current strategies for primary prevention of allergy

The Nutritional Committees of the American Academy of Paediatrics (AAP), the European Society for Paediatric Allergology and Clinical Immunology (ESPACI) and the European Society for Paediatric Gastroenterology, Hepatology and Nutrition (ESPGHAN) have prepared guidelines for the primary prevention of allergic diseases through dietary manipulation of expectant mothers and infants.[28, 29] These are slightly discrepant, being based on emerging evidence. The principal recommendations of these sets of guidelines are summarized in Table 2.

Probiotics are non-pathogenic Lactobacilli which enhance immune responses. The gut of newborn infants becomes colonized very quickly with up to 10 billion non-pathogenic micro-organisms soon after birth. This is probably a major source of immune stimulation. Researchers have sought to enhance this stimulation by feeding infants or their breast-feeding mothers with Lactobacilli, which protect against gut infections and may inhibit Th2 T cell responses. Early data[30] are encouraging, but more work needs to be done before this practice can be recommended routinely.

Although allergens are transmitted to the developing foetus through the placenta,[24] studies have failed to show that maternal avoidance of highly allergenic foods such as milk and egg alter the numbers of "at-risk" infants developing allergic disease if they are fed hypoallergenic diets after birth.[31] It is questionable whether such complete avoidance is possible.

Many food allergens eaten by lactating mothers are found intact in breast milk. Despite the theoretical risk that this may increase sensitization of infants to foodstuffs, two meta-analyses[32,33] of investigator blinded, prospective studies showed on the contrary a protective effect on breast-feeding on the development of eczema and asthma, but only in "at-risk" infants. The mechanism is unknown, but

Table 2. Approaches to primary prevention of allergy based on AAP and ESPACI/ESPGHAN guidelines*

Intervention	Comments
Probiotics in infant feed or during pregnancy/lactation	Experimental and not yet recommended
Dietary manipulation in pregnancy	Not recommended as not shown to be beneficial, although avoidance of nuts is easy and can do no harm
Dietary manipulation during breast-feeding	Not recommended since evidence of efficacy conflicting; again nuts are easy to avoid; total avoidance of eggs and cow's milk is virtually impossible and may result in maternal malnutrition
Breast-feeding	Exclusive breast-feeding recommended for 4–6 months
Soya formulae	Not recommended since no evidence for a protective effect against allergic disease in the child
Hypoallergenic formula for exclusive bottle-feeding or supplementation	Recommended. There is greater support for a beneficial effect of extensively hydrolysed formula, but its expense and unpalatability will limit its use.
Delayed introduction of solid foods to the infant	Start at 6 months of age. If possible, avoid cow's milk for at least 12 months; in highly motivated families, AAP recommends avoidance of eggs until 24 months and nuts and fish until 36 months.

*Measures generally effective for "at risk" children only (see text).

is one more reason to recommend breast-feeding in all infants so far as this is possible.

A Cochrane meta-analysis[34] of trials of maternal dietary avoidance of egg, milk and fish during breast-feeding noted some protective effect against the development of atopic dermatitis in the fed infants, but also noted that the number of studies was too small to consider the conclusion definitive. For this reason, maternal dietary manipulation during breast-feeding is not currently recommended.

Soya formulae do not prevent the development of atopy[35] and may pose risks associated with their phytoestrogen content.[36] They are not recommended specifically for the purpose of allergy prevention. 15% of infants allergic to cow's milk are also allergic to soya.

There is accumulating evidence that feeding with hydrolysed milk formulae reduces the risk of atopic disease in children.[37, 38] For this reason the use of such formulae for "at-risk" infants, either exclusively or as a supplement to breast milk, is recommended. There is some evidence that delayed introduction of solid foods until 4–6 months of life is similarly protective.[39]

Asthma

Definition

Despite decades of research, it has not been possible to define asthma purely in terms of histopathological features. Abnormal function of the airways remains inherent in the diagnosis, and although airways inflammation is a universal feature of asthma, the precise relationship between this inflammation and the functional abnormalities of the airways is still very poorly understood. A definition of asthma therefore encompasses:

- Inflammation of the airways: eosinophil influx orchestrated by Th2 type cytokines released by T cells (at least some allergen-specific) is usual, but not always prominent. Mucosal damage by eosinophils and cytokines (see earlier section) is thought to cause airways dysfunction.
- Variable airways obstruction: varies from none to severe in the course of hours to minutes, and is reversible both spontaneously and after suitable therapy.
- Non-specific hyper-reactivity: refers to the tendency of asthmatic airways to constrict in response to a wide variety of non-specific stimuli (including strong smells, cold air, fog, smoke, exercise, aerosol sprays, dust), which would not cause significant obstruction in non-asthmatics. This is again thought to be a consequence of airways inflammation, but the precise mechanisms are not clear.

Diagnosis

The cardinal clinical features of asthma are those of obstruction (wheeze, chest tightness, shortness of breath) and hyper-reactivity of the airways (wheeze in response to non-specific stimuli, cough). Any one of these symptoms may present in isolation. Symptoms of asthma may show diurnal variability (worse in the early hours of the morning), so it is important when making the diagnosis to ask patients specifically about day, night and early morning symptoms. It is quite common to find no physical signs at all on physical examination, although if airways obstruction is severe enough there may be diffuse, expiratory wheeze on auscultation. Additional clinical signs in the chest and/or an abnormal chest x-ray suggest an alternative or additional diagnosis (Table 3). These patients should be referred for specialist investigation.

Table 3. Diagnoses that may masquerade as asthma

Children	Adults	As part of the asthmatic diathesis
Diagnosis	**Diagnosis**	**Diagnosis**
Obliterative bronchiolitis	Cystic fibrosis	Allergic bronchopulmonary aspergillosis
Vocal cord dysfunction	Bronchiectasis	Pulmonary eosinophilic syndromes (e.g. Churg-Strauss)
Bronchomalacia	Inhaled foreign body	
Inhaled foreign bodies	Tracheobronchomalacia	
Cystic fibrosis	Recurrent aspiration	
Recent aspiration (particularly in handicapped children)	Chronic obstructive pulmonary disease	
Developmental abnormalities of the upper airway	Congestive cardiac failure	
Immunoglobulin deficiencies	Tumours in or impinging on central airways	
Primary ciliary dyskinesia	Obstructive bronchiolitis	
	Vocal cord dysfunction	
	Bronchial amyloidosis	
Signs	**Signs**	**Signs**
Persistent productive cough	Crackles in the chest	Involvement of other organs in vasculitis
Excessive vomiting	Evidence of heart failure	
Dysphagia	Unilateral or fixed wheeze	
Abnormality of the voice/cry	Stridor	
Failure to thrive	Persistent chest pain	
Focal signs in the chest	Productive cough	
	Weight loss	
	Non-resolving pneumonia	

Table 4. Objective criteria for diagnosis of asthma* (any of these features is diagnostic)

- \> 20% diurnal variability for more than 3 days/week for 2 weeks in a PEF diary

- Increase in FEV1 or PEF ≥ 15% after short-acting β_2-agonist or course of oral steroids

- Fall in FEV1 or PEF ≥ 15% after a 6-minute run (children)

- Positive histamine or methacholine challenge test (occasionally needed in difficult cases)

*Based on BTS/SIGN criteria. British Guideline on the Management of Asthma. *Thorax* 2003; **58** (Suppl. 1): i1–94.

It is very important to document the diagnosis of asthma objectively. This is usually based on simple spirometric measurements made in the surgery or clinic, or on home PEF measurements made in a diary (Table 4). A useful diagnostic test in children is to ask them to run vigorously for 6 minutes. The "gold standard" of asthma diagnosis is the histamine or methacholine challenge test (performed in hospital laboratories). Although this is a very sensitive and discriminating test, it is rarely needed to diagnose asthma. It is occasionally useful in cases where the diagnosis is in doubt, for example in patients with chronic cough whose peak flow variability is not quite diagnostic of asthma.

In children, the diagnosis of asthma may be more difficult, particularly in those children not old enough to perform spirometry reliably. In such cases, diagnosis rests on a suggestive history of typical symptoms, daily variability of these symptoms and the presence of characteristic exacerbating factors. Ultimately, the diagnosis may depend on a good response to a trial of anti-asthma therapy. A poor response should prompt careful review of the diagnosis. However the diagnosis is made, this should always be documented clearly in the patient's records.

Pharmacological therapy

In the UK, new guidelines have recently been published by the British Thoracic Society (BTS) in collaboration with the Scottish Intercollegiate Guidelines Network (SIGN).[40] The evidence tables on which these guidelines have been based are available on the website www.sign.ac.uk/guidelines/published/support/guideline63/download.html . Others have been issued by other bodies such as the Global Initiative for Asthma (GINA: www.ginasthma.com). The advantage of such guidelines is that they attempt to rationalize therapy, hopefully based on properly designed clinical trials. A disadvantage is that they tend to discourage consideration of the hopes, fears, aspirations, disease patterns and exacerbating factors in each individual patient. This is necessary for effective management.

Anti-asthma therapy is designed to address the two main pathophysiological entities associated with asthma, namely inflammation of the airways and inappropriate airways constriction. To reduce inflammation of the airways, the cornerstone of therapy is treatment with a topical glucocorticoid delivered by aerosol or dry powder inhalers. These must be taken regularly to control airways inflammation. They are referred to as "preventer" therapy to help the patient understand that they must be taken regularly, even in the absence of symptoms, in order to control asthmatic inflammation. To control inappropriate bronchospasm, both short-acting and long-acting β_2-agonists are used. These are referred to as "relievers".

The management of asthma is in adults and children is summarized in Table 5. Although this "stepwise" approach implies tailoring of treatment to suit symptoms, in practice it is usual to over treat patients initially, especially if they have severe symptoms. This promotes confidence in the treatment because the patient can usually sense a rapid improvement. After this, it is important to consider "stepping down" if the patient has remained stable for a considerable period: the BTS/SIGN guidelines suggest

Table 5. Stepwise management of asthma

Adults and children >12 years of age	Children 5–12 years of age	Children < 5 years of age
Step 1: Mild intermittent asthma: "as required" reliever therapy		
Inhaled SABA as required	Inhaled SABA as required	Inhaled SABA as required
Step 2: Regular preventer therapy		
Add inhaled steroid 200–800 µg/day*	Add inhaled steroid 200–400 µg/day*	Add inhaled steroid 200–400 µg/day*
Step 3: Add-on therapies		
Add inhaled LABA: • If good response, continue • If partial but inadequate response, continue LABA and increase inhaled steroids up to 800 µg/day* • If no response, stop LABA, increase inhaled steroids and consider other therapies such LTRA, SR theophylline	Add inhaled LABA: • If good response, continue • If partial but inadequate response, continue LABA and increase inhaled steroids up to 400 µg/day* • If no response, stop LABA, increase inhaled steroids and consider other therapies such LTRA, SR theophylline	In children aged between 2 and 5 years, consider addition of LTRA In children under 2 years, consider proceeding to Step 4
Step 4: Persistent poor control		
Increase inhaled steroid up to 2000 µg/day* Consider adding additional drug such as LTRA, SR theophylline	Increase inhaled steroid up to 800 µg/day*	Increase inhaled steroid up to 800 µg/day* Refer for specialist care
Step 5: Continuous oral steroids		
Daily steroid tablets, maintain high dosage inhaled steroids, refer for specialist care	Daily steroid tablets, maintain high dosage inhaled steroids, refer for specialist care	Refer for specialist care

SABA = short-acting β_2-agonist; LABA = long-acting β_2-agonist;
LTRA = leukotriene-receptor antagonist; SR = slow release.
*Refers to beclometasone or budesonide; equivalent dosages for fluticasone should be halved since clinically this is twice as potent.

reduction of inhaled steroids by 25–50% every 3 months if disease remains well controlled.

In patients at steps 1–3 of the treatment guidelines, it is reasonable to aim for perfect asthma control. This means that the patient should experience minimal symptoms, both day and night, have minimal need for reliever medication and no disease exacerbations, should experience no limitation of physical activity and should have normal lung function (FEV_1 or PEF > 80% of the predicted value). In those patients who continue to have severe troublesome symptoms despite maximum step 3 therapy, perfect asthma control is not a realistic aim, and in these cases it is a question of balancing the requirements of a reasonable quality of life against the risks of excessive high dose steroid medication. The patient's view should be taken into account when making such choices.

In the UK, approximately 85% of patients have mild disease controllable at steps 1, 2 or 3 of medication. These patients are managed largely in primary care and rarely need to visit hospital. The remaining 15% of patients have more severe, persistent symptoms (steps 4 or 5), and often require regular review by a hospital specialist. These patients are also more likely also to require hospital admission.

Steps 1–3

Patients with very mild symptoms may take a short-acting β_2-agonist when required. Daily symptoms requiring a puff of reliever or imperfect spirometry (see earlier) necessitate regular preventer therapy with inhaled steroids.

There are four inhaled steroids currently available for asthma therapy in the UK, beclometasone, budesonide, fluticasone and the recently introduced mometasone. Both fluticasone and mometasone are clinically more potent than beclometasone and budesonide, and as a rule of thumb they are as clinically effective as twice the dosages of these latter drugs. Inhaled steroids, if used at daily dosages below 800 µg/day (400 µg/day in children), are extremely safe. The only commonly encountered problem is local effects on the larynx, where they may cause hoarseness of the voice and local thrush infection. At such dosages, there is little to choose between the available steroid preparations. Where high dosages of inhaled steroids are necessary at step 3 and above, the decreased bioavailability of fluticasone and the mometasone coupled with their increased local potency may offer a more favourable benefit/risk ratio. One clear product of asthma research in the last few years has been a demonstration that early addition of a regular long-acting β_2-agonist (salmeterol and formoterol are currently available in the UK) exerts a steroid-sparing effect in asthmatics inadequately controlled at step 3 and also results in fewer symptoms and disease exacerbations.[41,42] For this reason, inhalers are now available which combine a fixed dosage of long-acting β_2-agonist with variable dosages of inhaled steroid. These preparations are convenient for the patient, may encourage compliance and save patients money if they have to pay for their own prescriptions.

Leukotrienes are produced by a wide variety of inflammatory cells, and in particular eosinophils and mast cells (see previous section). They are the most potent natural bronchoconstrictors known, and also increase mucus secretion and promote vascular leakage. The leukotriene-receptor antagonists montelukast and zafirlukast have been shown to improve lung function and symptoms, and reduce disease exacerbation.[43,44] Because the response to these drugs is less predictable, they are not used as first-line therapy at step 3, but may be useful adjuncts to therapy (this should preferably be documented by peak expiratory flow [PEF] monitoring). Theophyllines inhibit the enzyme phosphodiesterase, leading to increased intracellular concentrations of cyclic AMP, which relaxes bronchial smooth muscle and inhibits inflammatory cells. These effects are however weak and, in addition, theophyllines more frequently cause troublesome unwanted effects. Addition of inhaled anticholinergics at this stage is generally of no value, while cromoglycate and nedocromil confer only marginal benefit.

Step 4

There are no clear guidelines as to the best course of treatment for Step 4 patients. Options include increasing inhaled steroids up to 2,000 µg/day (adults) or 800 µg/day (children), or adding in a leukotriene receptor antagonist, oral theophylline or oral slow release β_2-agonist. Inhaled steroid dosages should not be increased over these limits; this has led to adrenal crisis on rapid withdrawal in children. Drugs should be altered one at a time, with monitoring of efficacy, and discontinued if not objectively effective. Patients still struggling with symptoms at this stage, especially children, should be considered for referral for specialist care.

Step 5

If patients are deemed to require steroid tablets long-term, maximal dosages of inhaled steroid and other add-on therapy *if shown to be effective* should be continued. Inhaled steroids are the most effective drugs for minimizing the requirement for oral steroids.[45,46] Patients on regular oral steroids should be monitored (and treated if practicable) for the development of:

- Hypertension
- Diabetes mellitus
- Osteoporosis (see guidelines of the National Osteoporosis Society www.nos.org.uk)
- Poor growth and cataract in children.

Adults and children at steps 4 and 5 should be considered for specialist referral.

Why isn't my patient responding?

The important factors which may contribute to reduce the maximal potential response of patients to therapy are summarized in Table 6. Obviously, it is important to make *and document* the correct diagnosis, as described above, and increase dosages of therapy if insufficient.

Technique and understanding

Incorrect inhaler technique is common: one overview[47] suggests that 50% of patients do not know how to use their inhalers correctly, and that this is improved by training.

Table 6. Why isn't my patient responding?
• Incorrect or additional diagnosis • Inadequate dosages of therapy • Poor patient compliance or understanding • Allergen exposure • Exercise-induced asthma • Allergic bronchopulmonary aspergillosis • Drugs: β-blockers, aspirin/NSAIDS • Smoking (active or passive) • Occupational disease • Hormonal: pre-menstrual asthma, hypothyroidsism • Underlying vasculitis (Churg-Strauss syndrome) • True steroid refractoriness/resistance

Patients must also clearly understand the necessity for regular preventer therapy, even when the disease is well controlled. Many inhaler devices are now available, and there are few clear indications that they differ in their effectiveness, but some patients prefer dry powder devices to metered dose (propellant) inhalers. Steroid inhalers should always be used with a spacer (and a face mask in infants). Spacers should be washed monthly with soap and water and renewed at least yearly. There is no evidence that nebulized steroids are more effective than a metered dose inhaler and spacer when treating chronic asthma. In primary care, asthmatics should be reviewed regularly by a nurse with training in asthma management. Clinical review should be proactive and empower individuals or their parents/carers to undertake self-management effectively. Such review should include:

- Measurement of lung function (PEF)
- Inhaler technique
- Morbidity (for example as assessed by the Royal College of Physicians' "three questions"[48]):
  - Have you had difficulty sleeping because of asthma?
  - Have you had your usual asthma symptoms during the day?
  - Has your asthma interfered with your usual activities?

- Current treatment
- Asthma action plan (all patients in step 3 and above, and all those who have had a severe exacerbation in the past year, should have an asthma action plan). Plans should be focused on individual needs and may be based on symptoms and/or PEF measurements, depending on patient ability. They have been shown to improve health outcomes.[49-52] A number of model plans is available from the National Asthma Campaign www.asthma.org.uk/control.

Allergen exposure

Exposure to aeroallergens clearly exacerbates asthma[53-55] and increases the risk of acute exacerbations[56] in allergic individuals, and no assessment of asthma is complete without assessment by an allergist. Clinical suspicion of sensitivity to particular allergens should be backed up by skin prick testing or RAST. House dust mite allergy is an important trigger in perennial asthma. Asthmatic symptoms related to animal dander are easily identified. Allergy to the moulds *Alternaria* or *Cladosporium* may be an important cause of severe seasonal asthma in the late summer and autumn, or perennial asthma in damp and mouldy homes. Inquiry should specifically be made about allergens to which the patients may be sensitized in their own homes. Atopic patients often have concomitant allergic rhinitis, which should always be treated, usually with topical nasal steroids. Although many experts feel that removal of pets from the homes of individuals with asthma who show IgE-mediated clinical sensitivity should be recommended, it has been difficult to obtain evidence that allergen avoidance in the population as a whole plays a role in asthma management. This, in part, reflects the impracticability of performing blinded trials, and may also reflect the fact that clinically relevant avoidance of many allergens (pollens, moulds, house dust mite) is impossible. Two Cochrane reviews[57,58] addressing house dust mite avoidance concluded that current clinical and physical methods of dust mite eradication are ineffective, while physical barrier methods (particularly complete barrier bed covering systems) showed marginal benefit. IgE-mediated sensitization to *Aspergillus* suggests the possibility of allergic bronchopulmonary aspergillosis. If this is confirmed by other investigations, a 4-month trial of itraconazole should be considered in patients with severe symptoms taking oral steroids.

Some 30–40% of asthmatics, particularly adults with late onset disease, are non-atopic. It is equally important to demonstrate the lack of allergic sensitization in these patients, where allergen avoidance is not known to be appropriate.

Specific allergen immunotherapy is widely used for the management of appropriately sensitized atopic asthmatics in Europe and the USA. Three meta-analyses[59-61] addressing immunotherapy with various allergens have shown benefit as compared with placebo, particularly with allergen-induced symptoms and increased bronchial hyper-reactivity. There is also some evidence that it may alter the natural history of asthma, reducing the onset of new allergic sensitization.[62] This practice is not, however, currently recommended for the management of atopic asthma in the UK by the British Society for Allergy and Clinical Immunology (BSACI) or the BTS, since asthmatics are much more susceptible to the acute effects of anaphylaxis, and also because the possible benefits of allergen immunotherapy in reducing or substituting for conventional pharmacological therapy have never been properly assessed.

Drugs: β-blockers and aspirin

β-Blockers, including eye drops, are contraindicated in asthmatics since they may cause acute, severe bronchospasm. Aspirin-sensitive patients may develop one or more of a constellation of symptoms (bronchospasm, rhinitis, gastrointestinal upset, urticaria) acutely following aspirin ingestion. Aspirin sensitivity is seen in about 10% of adult asthmatics, and is usually diagnosed by a careful clinical history of suggestive symptoms developing within minutes or hours of aspirin ingestion. This effect reflects the ability of aspirin and related non-steroidal anti-inflammatory drugs (NSAIDs) to inhibit the cyclo-oxygenase isoenzyme COX-1, which mediates the formation of prostaglandins, some of which (such as PGE_2) may be protective against bronchospasm. Aspirin-sensitive asthmatics must assiduously avoid aspirin and other COX-1 inhibitors, but it is not automatically logical to ban all asthmatics from using these drugs, particularly if indicated for valid therapeutic purposes. In cases of doubt, the patient should be referred to an allergist for formal aspirin challenge. Since the effects of aspirin are metabolic rather than IgE-mediated, aspirin-sensitivity cannot be diagnosed by skin prick testing or RAST. Increasing evidence suggests that newer anti-inflammatory drugs such as rofecoxib, which inhibit the distinct cyclo-oxygenase isoenzyme COX-2, may be safe in aspirin-sensitive patients. It is important to remember, however, that these drugs do not substitute for the anti-platelet effects of aspirin.

Smoking

Maternal smoking in pregnancy has an adverse effect on lung development[63] and may increase the risk of allergic sensitisation of the offspring.[64] Exposure to environmental tobacco smoke (passive smoking) increases the risk of asthma exacerbation in children.[65] Starting smoking in a teenager increases the risk of persisting asthma.[66] It is unclear as yet whether smoking in adults increases symptoms or exacerbations. Nevertheless, for all these reasons smoking should be discouraged.

Occupational asthma

Occupational asthma may now account for up to 10% of cases of adult onset asthma. The diagnosis should be suspected and sought in all adult asthmatics, particularly those in high-risk occupations. Patients should be asked if their symptoms are better when away from work or on holiday. Serial PEF measurements every 2 hours whilst at home and at work, from waking to sleeping, may suggest the diagnosis: analysis is best done with the aid of a criterion-based expert system (see www.occupationalasthma.com). The precise cause is a best sought by an occupational physician. Most, but not all patients show evidence of IgE-mediated sensitization to the offending agent (common examples include latex, flour, enzymes, rodent urine extracts and animal dander). The prognosis is worse for workers who develop occupational asthma and remain exposed to the offending agent for more than 1 year after symptoms develop.[67] Management options include removing the cause from the workplace, or moving the employee to an alternative job.

Alternative and complementary medicine

This is discussed in more detail in the BTS/SIGN guidelines[40] but, briefly, at present there is no clear evidence-based confirmation that herbal medicine, acupuncture, air ionizers, homoeopathy, chiropractic or breathing exercises, including yoga and Buteyko, improve asthma objectively, although some of these alternatives may discourage inappropriate over-breathing associated with anxiety.

Management of acute, severe asthma

An account of this is beyond the scope of this book. Full guidelines, however, for the management of acute asthma in both adults and children are provided in the BTS/SIGN guideline.[40]

Allergic rhinitis and conjunctivitis

Introduction

Non-infectious rhinitis, commonly associated with allergy, is one of the commonest diseases worldwide, resulting in considerable morbidity for millions of people. It is a disease of young patients, starting from pre-school age to middle-age. It is unusual for allergic rhinitis to commence in patients older than 50 years.

In the large International Study of Asthma and Allergies in Childhood (ISAAC) on the incidence of allergic in diseases in children worldwide,[68] the prevalence of allergic rhinitis varied geographically from 1% to 40%. The prevalence of allergic rhinitis in "developed" countries was relatively high at 15–20%. A similar prevalence was observed in a Swiss study.[69] In most Western countries, the incidence of allergic rhinitis has shown an alarming and dramatic increase.

Aetiology

1. *Allergen-specific T cell responses.* Non-infectious rhinitis is probably initiated by a Th2-type T cell response to allergens (see *Definition, pathogenesis and epidemiology*). Cytokines and chemokines are produced locally, causing eosinophils and mast cell influx into the nasal mucosa. This causes chronic hypertrophy of the mucosa and the symptom of nasal blockage, and may result in local tissue remodelling (such as nasal polyps). Chronic blockage may impair the sensations of taste and smell. This process is inhibited by steroids but not by antihistamines.

2. *Allergen-specific IgE.* Most, but not all, patients with rhinitis also produce allergen-specific IgE and have

IgE-sensitized mast cells in the nasal mucosa. On exposure to allergens, mast cells degranulate, producing acute sneezing, itching and clear rhinorrhoea. The timing of these symptoms depends on the spectrum of allergens to which the patient is clinically sensitized.

3. *Mediators.* Eosinophils produce granule proteins and cysteinyl leukotrienes, which respectively damage the nasal mucosa and cause local oedema. Histamine irritates local nerve afferents causing sneeze and itch, amplified by other mast cell mediators (tryptase, prostaglandins and leukotrienes), which also increase mucus secretion and attract further inflammatory cells.

4. *Abnormality of the target organ.* Not all patients sensitized to inhaled aeroallergens develop rhinitis, and rhinitis can occur in the absence of allergen-specific IgE responses. This suggests that there may be some abnormality of the nasal mucosa (possibly genetic, acted on by environmental factors), which allows rhinitis to develop in some subjects but not others (see also *Definition, pathogenesis and epidemiology*).

Clinical features

The principal features of chronic rhinitis are nasal blockage, sneezing, itching of the nose, throat and ears, rhinorrhoea and loss of taste and smell. In non-allergic rhinitis, blockage predominates. In allergic rhinitis, the manifestation of additional symptoms (sneeze, itch, rhinorrhoea) will depend on allergen exposure, which has resulted in the traditional classification of allergic rhinitis into seasonal (implying clinical sensitization to allergens present at a particular season of the year) or perennial (allergens present all the year round). In the recent World Health Organization Initiative on Allergic Rhinitis and its Impact on Asthma (ARIA),[70] it was suggested that allergic rhinitis should be re-classified as "intermittent" or "persistent", in recognition of the fact that some individuals may be intermittently exposed to perennial allergens. A list of the common

Table 7. Principal aeroallergens that may exacerbate allergic rhinitis	
Allergen	**Timing of symptoms**
• **House dust mite** Dermatophagoides, Euroglyphus	Persistent
• **Other mites** Glycyphagus, Tyrophagus (stocked grains), Panonychus (apple and citrus trees), Ornithonyssus (poultry breeders)	Intermittent
• **Animals** Cat, dog, horse, cow, rabbit, mouse, rat (allergens in skin glands, saliva, urine)	Intermittent or persistent
• **Tree pollens** Birch, alder, hazel, ash, oak, plane	Intermittent (February–May)
• **Grass pollens**	Intermittent (May–July)
• **Weed pollens** Mugwort, ragweed	Intermittent (July–September)
• **Mould (fungal) spores** Cladosporium, Alternaria Penicillium, Aspergillus	Intermittent (summer) if exposure occurs outside; persistent if the fungi grow in damp houses
• **Occupational agents** High-molecular weight (allergens which produce an IgE response) – latex, laboratory animals, flour, coffee, enzymes, wood dust and many others	Intermittent or persistent
Low-molecular weight (sensitizers that do not produce an IgE response) – isocyanates, aldehydes and many others	Intermittent or persistent

aeroallergens which may exacerbate allergic rhinitis is shown in Table 7. In addition, it is important to remember that acute exacerbations of rhinitis may be a manifestation of food allergies (principally cow's milk, egg, soya and nuts) in infants and young children.

Table 8. Comparison of major clinical features of seasonal/intermittent rhinitis and perennial/persistent allergic rhinitis		
Clinical feature	Seasonal/intermittent	Perennial/persistent
Nasal obstruction	Variable	Universal, marked
Nasal secretion	Common, watery	Variable, seromucous, post-nasal drip
Sneezing	Prominent	Variable
Disturbance of taste and smell	Variable	Common
Associated eye symptoms	Common	Unusual
Associated asthma	Variable	Common
Chronic sinusitis	Occasional	Frequent

Different features of the disease tend to predominate in seasonal/intermittent rhinitis as compared with perennial/persistent disease, as shown in Table 8.[71]

Comorbidity

Chronic rhinosinusitis, whether allergic or non-allergic, is frequently associated with asthma, and there is increasing realization that patients with asthma may have at least some sub-clinical inflammatory changes in the nasal mucosa, and *vice versa*.[71] Epidemiological studies have clearly confirmed that rhinitis is a risk factor for asthma.[72] Conversely, in a retrospective study of patients with rhinitis and asthma,[73] patients receiving regular anti-inflammatory therapy (topical steroids) for rhinitis were less likely to present with acute exacerbations of asthma. It is therefore of critical importance to consider a possible diagnosis of asthma in patients with rhinitis, and *vice versa*, and to investigate and treat both diseases appropriately. Allergic conjunctivitis commonly occurs in association with allergic rhinitis, whether intermittent or persistent. Allergen avoidance measures in patients with asthma, rhinitis and conjunctivitis should embrace, where possible, all three diseases.

Chronic nasal congestion from untreated allergic rhinitis may result in obstruction of the sinus ostia and secondary bacterial infection, resulting in acute bacterial sinusitis. Further obstruction leads to low oxygen tension,

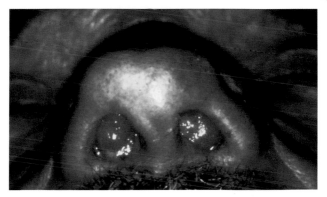

Figure 6. Severe bilateral nasal polyposis with complete obstruction of the nasal cavity. Reproduced with permission from Corrigan C, Klimek L, Hörmann K. *Rhinitis: Illustrated Differential Diagnosis.* London: Mosby. 2001.

predisposing to anaerobic infection. This may cause mucopurulent postnasal drip, facial pain and headache.

Nasal polyps may result from chronic inflammation (often allergic) of the nasal mucosa, and prolapse into the middle meatus and are visible as translucent, insensitive swellings (Figure 6). They further exacerbate blockage and cause headache, facial pain and secondary infection. They are common in aspirin-sensitive patients, who may have associated asthma and urticaria. Polyps are very rare in children, where they are usually caused by cystic fibrosis or meningocoele (see *Differential diagnosis* below).

Psychosocial morbidity in allergic rhinitis is enormous and often trivialized by non-sufferers. Severe intermittent rhinitis, such as hayfever, reduces attention span and intellectual ability, as well as self-esteem and image.[74] It is one of the commonest causes of loss and time from school and work, with enormous economic implications.

Differential diagnosis

The causes of rhinitis are listed in Table 9. Most causes are infective or allergic. Rarely, chronic bacterial or fungal

Table 9. Causes of rhinitis

Allergic			Infective		Structural	Other causes	
Seasonal allergens	Perennial allergens	Occupational allergens	Acute rhinitis	Chronic rhinitis		Local	Systemic
Tree Grass Weeds Moulds	House dust mite Animals Moulds	High-molecular weight - Latex - Laboratory animals - Grains - Wood dusts Low-molecular weight - Isocyanates - Aldehydes - Platinum - Salts	Viral infection Bacterial infection	Bacterial infection Unusual causes - Anaerobes - Tuberculosis - Leprosy - Rhinosderoma - Yaws - Glanders Fungal - Rhinosporidiosis - Cryptococcosis - Aspergillosis - Blastomycosis - Histoplasmosis - Sporotrichosis - Candidiasis	Polyps Deviated nasal septum Hypertrophy of inferior turbinates Enlarged adenoids Anatomical variants Foreign body Choanal atresia	Idiopathic rhinitis Non-allergic rhinitis Drug-induced rhinitis - β-blockers - oral contraceptives - hormone replacement therapy - aspirin and NSAIDs - topical nasal decongestants Neoplastic rhinitis	Mucous abnormality - cystic fibrosis - Young's syndrome Ciliary abnormality - primary ciliary dyskinesia - Kartagener's syndrome Immune Deficiency - Ig deficiency - HIV-related Connective tissue disorders - SLE - Sjögren's syndrome - systemic sclerosis Granulomatous disorders - Wegener's granulomatosis - sarcoidosis Hormonal - lack of thyroxine - growth hormone excess - pregnancy
Intermittent symptoms < 4 days/week or for < 4 weeks		Persistent symptoms > 4 days/week and for at least 4 weeks					

infections may be responsible for chronic rhinosinusitis. Anatomical abnormalities may occur alone or as a result of untreated chronic inflammation. Rhinitis may be caused or exacerbated by drugs, particularly β-blockers, oestrogens, and aspirin and related drugs in sensitive patients. Chronic bacterial rhinosinusitis may be a feature of cystic fibrosis, cilliary abnormalities or immunoglobulin deficiency syndromes. The nasal mucosa may also be involved in connective tissue diseases and granulomatous disorders. Very rarely, cerebrospinal fluid leakage may occur into the nasal cavity and mimic chronic rhinorrhoea.

Diagnosis

Clinical history and examination

As always, a careful clinical history is the key to correct diagnosis. Symptoms of nasal blockage, running nose, itching and sneezing, and loss of sense of taste or smell should be specifically sought. If symptoms are intermittent, it is important to establish their temporal relationship to known sources of allergens (Table 7). Many patients have persistent symptoms with seasonal exacerbations. Acute symptoms are less prominent in persistent/perennial disease (Table 8). With rhinitis caused by perennial allergens such as house dust mite, it is often difficult to relate symptoms clearly to allergen exposure (although since most mite exposure occurs in bed, patients may have nocturnal and early morning symptoms). All patients with persistent nasal blockage and discharge should be assumed to have persistent allergic rhinitis until proven otherwise. Enquiry should also be made about comorbid conditions (asthma, sinusitis, conjunctivitis and eczema). The possibility that symptoms may be drug- or work-related should be considered. In infants and children, the possibility that food allergies may be causing symptoms should be considered, as should the possibility of congenital disorders such as cystic fibrosis.

Fixed, unilateral nasal blockage is usually the result of a structural abnormality such as a deviated nasal septum or, more rarely, a foreign body or a tumour. The principal causes of nasal blockage and discharge in the absence of mechanical blockage are allergic and infective rhinitis. These should be easy to distinguish from a careful history, but it is surprising how often persistent allergic rhinitis is confused with a "cold that will not go away".

Nasal problems are often multifactorial. For example, untreated allergic rhinitis may result in secondary sinus obstruction and bacterial sinusitis, which is further exacerbated by a nasal structural abnormality. It is essential to treat the underlying cause as well as the end result. Simple clinical examination may reveal nasal blockage, polyps and nasal septal deviation, but more complex problems require the expertise of an ENT specialist.

Investigations

Suspected allergenic causes of rhinitis derived from the history should be confirmed with skin prick testing or RAST. A suitable list of possible aeroallergens for skin prick testing is shown in Table 7. As always, positive skin prick tests have a poor positive predictive value for clinical symptoms, and so the significance of positive skin prick tests can only be interpreted in the light of a clear history of exposure to the allergen causing symptoms. Large molecular weight occupational allergens producing an IgE response can be investigated with skin prick test or RAST, but smaller molecular weight molecules, which do not produce such a response, require specific challenge procedures, usually under the guidance of an occupational physician. Some patients with persistent rhinitis have uniformly negative skin prick tests; in the absence of any other possible cause (Table 9), these patients can be assumed to have non-atopic rhinitis, which is essentially a diagnosis of exclusion. Patients with suspected underlying systemic diseases should have these investigated in their own right.

Management

Avoidance

Where practical, the patient should be advised about avoidance of clinically relevant allergens. Pollen is impossible to avoid completely, but its exposure may be reduced by smearing petroleum jelly around the external nares to catch pollen, wearing "wrap around" sunglasses, closing windows in houses and cars and not using ventilators (unless pollen-filtered), avoiding heavy exercise outdoors and not going out in the evening when the air cools and the pollen falls to earth. Patients with animal allergy should not keep animals in their homes; even then, some allergens, particularly cat allergen, may take months to disappear, and the keeping of pets is now so widespread that cat and dog allergens are becoming ubiquitous. Dust mites thrive in warm, humid, poorly ventilated rooms in bedding and soft furnishings. Highly sensitized patients with marked nocturnal symptoms may derive some benefit from mite-impermeable bed coverings (mattress, duvet and pillows must all be covered). Allergens causing rhinitis and/or asthma in the work place must be strenuously avoided, since disease may become permanent even after removal of exposure.[75] This may involve alternative placement at work or even a change of job.

Pharmacotherapy

Non sedating antihistamines (cetirizine/levocetirizine, loratadine/desloratadine, acrivastine and fexofenadine) are safe and effective for mast cell-associated symptoms (rhinorrhoea, sneeze and itching), but less effective at reversing the T cell-mediated component of rhinitis (nasal blockage and loss of taste and smell). Many patients self-medicate with "over the counter" drugs. Regular, as opposed to intermittent, treatment is most effective. Topical nasal antihistamines (azelastine, levocabastine) used twice daily are also effective but do not affect associated conjunctivitis or itching elsewhere, and are not suitable when the nose is significantly blocked. Topical antihistamine eye drops are useful for associated conjunctivitis.

For mild-to-moderate disease, with significant nasal blockage, regular topical steroids are the treatment of choice. They have been clearly shown to reduce nasal blockage, rhinorrhoea and sneezing. They are more efficient in this regard than antihistamines. Patients must understand that they must be taken daily and regularly in a prophylactic fashion, and that they have little immediate effect on symptoms. For intermittent rhinitis caused by pollens, treatment should be commenced 2 or 3 weeks in advance of the start of the relevant pollen season. The correct inhaler technique must be demonstrated to the patient. Other topical steroids including budesonide, flunisolide, fluticasone and mometasone have joined beclometasone, the first available drug. The latter two drugs have the highest topical potency and relatively low bioavailability and therefore, perhaps, have a therapeutic edge although with all preparations, systemic effects are very rare. An exception is topical betametasone, which can exert systemic effects at high dosage: this drug is usually used for limited periods to treat severe blockage, especially with nasal polyps. Topical steroids may cause local crusting and minor epistaxis, especially when first used on a severely inflamed nasal mucosa. Perforation of the nasal septum is a rare complication of topical steroid therapy, often when excessive dosages are used with improper technique. Contact sensitivity to the excipients in some preparations is very rarely seen. Patients are often concerned that regular topical nasal steroid therapy will damage their nose; on the contrary, aside from the rare unwanted effects mentioned above, current findings suggest that regular topical nasal steroids, through their anti-inflammatory effect, promote resolution and repair of nasal mucosal damage.

Occasionally, short courses of oral steroids may be justified for very severe symptoms or prophylaxis during critical periods such as examinations.

Sodium cromoglycate and nedocromil sodium are available as topical therapy for allergic rhinitis and conjunctivitis. Although completely safe, they are less efficacious than antihistamines and topical steroids, and must be taken extremely frequently (more often then the recommended four times daily) to be effective.

Topical nasal decongestants (α1-agonists such as phenylephrine, α2-agonists such as oxymetazoline or xylometazoline or noradrenaline releasers such as ephedrine) are useful for short-term relief of nasal obstruction, for example prior to flying. Prolonged use causes rebound bogginess of the nasal mucosa (rhinitis medicamentosa). Topical ipratropium bromide, usually used in conjunction with anti-histamines and topical steroids, is occasionally used when troublesome rhinorrhoea predominates.

For children, some topical antihistamines may be used from 5 years, topical steroids from 6 years, and systemic antihistamines from 2 years. Avoidance of allergens, including food allergens, should be carefully investigated in children. Topical nasal steroids are safe in children, but there are occasions when they are avoided to reduce "total steroid load" in children already receiving inhaled steroids for asthma and topical steroid creams for eczema. Most manufacturers of non-sedating antihistamines recommend avoidance in pregnancy: chlorpheniramine is regarded as safe but is unfortunately sedating. Topical nasal steroids may safely be used in pregnancy, as may cromoglycate and nedocromil.

An excellent summary of the evidence regarding these recommendations may be found in the ARIA report.[70]

Allergen immunotherapy

Allergen immunotherapy is useful for the management of carefully selected patients with allergic rhinitis and conjunctivitis who have severe symptoms closely related to exposure to single allergens despite taking adequate pharmacotherapy. This is discussed fully in the section *Allergen immunotherapy*.

Surgical management

Surgical intervention for rhinitis is only rarely necessary, but may be needed for drug-resistant inferior turbinate hypertrophy, anatomical abnormalities of functional significance, secondary chronic sinusitis, including fungal sinusitis and advanced polyposis, tumours and cerebrospinal fluid leakage.

Atopic dermatitis

Atopic dermatitis is a disease that typically appears in early childhood and may have a profound effect on the lives of affected patients. As with all allergic diseases, there is evidence that the prevalence of atopic dermatitis has increased.[76] Currently, the lifetime prevalence of atopic dermatitis ranges from 10 to 20% in "developed" countries.[77] As with other atopic diseases, eczema tends to run in families and there is a particularly strong maternal influence.

Clinical features

The overriding clinical symptom of atopic dermatitis is pruritus or itch. Itch is usually much worse at night. Patients are sensitive to a wide variety of non-specific irritants such as wools, acrylic and soaps. In infancy, episodes of atopic dermatitis tend to be more acute, with intense excoriation of the skin, vesicles and serous exudates (Figure 7). In older children and adults, the disease tends to be more chronic with lichenification (Figure 8). In common with atopic diseases in general, the severity of atopic dermatitis seems to subside with age. Principal clinical features of atopic dermatitis are listed in Table 10.

Although atopic dermatitis presents a very typical clinical picture, there are some important differential diagnoses which must be considered and ruled out.

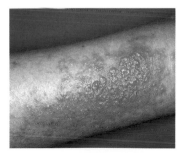

Figure 7. Acute eczema with marked erythema, superficial papulae and vesiculae, which easily excoriate and lead to crusts. Reproduced with permission from Holgate ST, Church MK, Lichtenstein LM. *Allergy. Second Edition*. London: Mosby. 2001.

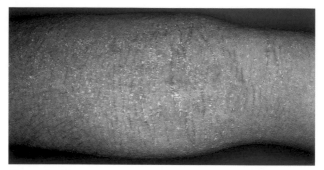

Figure 8. Chronic eczema characterized by faint erythema, infiltration and scaling. Reproduced with permission from Holgate ST, Church MK, Lichtenstein LM. *Allergy. Second Edition*. London: Mosby. 2001.

Table 10. Clinical features of atopic dermatitis (eczema)

- Pruritus (itch)
- Facial and extensor eczema in infants and children
- Flexural eczema in adults
- Chronic or relapsing dermatitis
- Elevated serum IgE and positive skin prick tests in 80% of patients
- Anterior subcapsular cataract
- Dennie-Morgan infra-orbital folds

Table 11. Differential diagnosis of atopic dermatitis (eczema)

- Congenital diseases: Netherton's syndrome, familial keratosis
- Chronic dermatoses: seborrhoeic dermatitis, psoriasis, icthyoses
- Infections: scabies, fungal infections
- Malignancies: mycosis fungoides, Letterer-Siwe disease
- Autoimmune disease: dermatomyositis
- Immunodeficiency: Wiskott-Aldrich syndrome, severe combined immunodeficiency, hyper-IgE syndrome
- Metabolic: zinc deficiency, pyridoxine deficiency, phenylketonuria

Certain congenital diseases (e.g. Netherton's syndrome, familial keratosis, congenital immune deficiencies such as Wiskott–Aldrich or hyper-IgE syndrome) would be suggested by the overall clinical picture and the family history. Occasionally, skin infestations such as scabies and fungal infections may be mistaken for atopic dermatitis.

Rarely, skin malignancies such as mycosis fungoides may superficially resemble atopic dermatitis. A list of the principal differential diagnoses to be considered is listed in Table 11.

Pathology

Atopic dermatitis, or eczema, is one of the triad of childhood atopic diseases. Most (80%), but not all patients, are atopic with elevated total and allergen-specific serum IgE concentrations. They typically have elevated circulating blood eosinophils and may have associated hayfever and asthma. As with other atopic diseases, an allergen-specific T cell response (with production of Th_2-type cytokines locally in the skin and consequent accumulation of granulocytes, particularly eosinophils) is thought to play an important part in the pathophysiology. Most patients with atopic dermatitis are sensitized to a variety of aeroallergens, and it is thought that sensitization occurs at least partly through the skin. In atopic, but not non-atopic, patients with dermatitis, allergen exposure may cause acute exacerbation of disease.

Trigger factors

Atopic dermatitis is a disease of exacerbation and remission, particularly in infants and younger children. The most important exacerbating factors include:

- Food allergens
- Aeroallergens
- Infection with *Staphylococcus aureus*.

The possibility of food allergy must always be considered in young children with atopic dermatitis.[78] 40% of infants and young children so affected have a food allergy, and removal of food allergens has been shown to produce significant clinical improvement. Typical allergens in infancy include eggs, milk, wheat, soya and nuts. Often, avoidance of these products can be complicated and requires expert dietary advice. Although positive skin prick tests to these food stuffs are consistent with a possibility of allergy, they are not necessarily associated with relevant clinical reactions to foods, which must be verified wherever possible by food challenge or an elimination diet. This requires assessment by an allergist.

It has been shown that the direct application of aeroallergens to unaffected skin of patients with atopic dermatitis induces erythematous reactions in up to 50% of patients.[79] Allergens which may do this include house dust mite, grass and weed pollens, animal dander and moulds. There is evidence[80-82] to suggest that efficient avoidance of house dust mite allergen in sensitized patients improves symptoms and severity of the disease. Again, allergy testing by skin prick test or RAST is an indispensable aspect of management.

Patients with atopic dermatitis have an increased tendency to develop skin infections with *Staphylococcus aureus* (Figure 9) and various viruses, in particular herpes simplex (Figure 10). Even patients without such obvious infections tend to respond better to topical steroids with antistaphylococcal antibiotics than steroids alone.[83] In addition to the local effects of infection, *Staphylococcus aureus* produces various toxins which act as superantigens, causing local activation

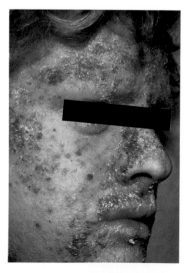

Figure 9. Atopic dermatitis secondarily infected with *Staphylococcus aureus*, and impetiginization of the face. Reproduced with permission from Holgate ST, Church MK, Lichtenstein LM. *Allergy. Second Edition*. London: Mosby. 2001.

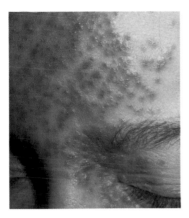

Figure 10. Atopic dermatitis secondarily infected with herpes simplex virus type I (eczema herpeticum). Reproduced with permission from Holgate ST, Church MK, Lichtenstein LM. *Allergy. Second Edition*. London: Mosby. 2001.

of subgroups of T cells. In addition, some patients produce IgE antibodies directed against these superantigens.

Management

This can be a very complicated process, and embraces not only pharmacological management of the disease, but also management of patients in terms of their lifestyle and morale. The cornerstones of medical management are adequate skin hydration, drug therapy and elimination of exacerbating factors. Ideally, treatment plans should be individualized to the skin reaction patterns of particular trigger factors of patients. In severe disease, immunomodulatory drugs may be administered (see Table 12 for a summary of atopic dermatitis management). A full list of topical therapies available is shown in Appendix 1.

Atopic dermatitis severely impairs the barrier function of the skin, causing water loss, xerosis, fissures and cracking. For this reason, patients must frequently hydrate the skin with baths and emollients. In addition, wet dressings enhance the penetration of topical steroids and discourage scratching.

Pharmacotherapy

It is very important to manage itch in patients with chronic atopic dermatitis. In part, this is be managed by reducing any underlying causes of the disease and minimizing

Table 12. Management of atopic dermatitis (eczema)

Mild/moderate disease	Severe disease

• Skin hydration/emollients
• Topical steroids
• Anti-histamines
• Topical calcineurin inhibitors (tacrolimus, pimecrolimus)
• Elimination of exacerbating factors
  - inhalant and food allergens
  - irritants
  - psychological
• Treatment of skin infections
	• Intensification of existing therapy
	• Hospitalization
	• Wet dressings
	• Systemic steroids
	• Cyclosporin
	• Phototherapy

exposure to trigger factors. Although many patients benefit from systemic antihistamines, this benefit is not evident in a proportion of patients, probably reflecting the fact that mediators other than histamine play a role in the pathogenesis of skin-itching. It is better to use non-sedating antihistamines, such as cetirizine, loratadine or fexofenadine during the day, although sedating antihistamines may be useful at night. Doxepin has both tricyclic antidepressant and histamine-receptor blocking activity: it may be useful for both of these properties in some patients. Topical antihistamine creams are not generally recommended since they may cause additional sensitization and local disease exacerbation.

Phototherapy is of some benefit in atopic dermatitis. Natural sunlight is very good for patients, but not if this is obtained in the context of high humidity and excessive sweating. Therapeutic broadband UVB, UVA and combined therapies can be useful adjuncts to treatment.[84] PUVA (combination of psoralen and long-wave UVA) therapy has been used for severe, widespread disease.

Short courses of systemic steroids may produce disease improvement, but there is often an associated rebound flare. Systemic steroid therapy for severe exacerbations of atopic dermatitis should always, therefore, be accompanied by intensification of direct skin care. Similarly, cyclosporin A therapy often produces temporary improvement, but there is a marked rebound of symptoms when it is withdrawn.

Traditionally, topical steroid creams have been used for acute exacerbations of disease, but are also increasingly used prophylactically (e.g. twice weekly application of fluticasone or mometasone[85]). In general, creams containing high-potency steroids should be avoided on the face and genitalia. For therapeutic purposes, cream should be applied only to skin lesions, although for prophylactic use it may be applied more extensively. Often, a large amount of cream may be needed: for example, 30 g may be needed to cover the entire skin surface of an average adult once over.

Topical steroids used for the treatment of atopic dermatitis are classified according to their potency. The unwanted effects of these preparations are similarly related to potency. Local unwanted effects include striae and skin atrophy. Systemic unwanted effects include suppression of the hypothalamic-pituitary-adrenal (HPA) axis, and occasionally other systemic effects such as hyperglycaemia and appetite stimulation. The risk of these effects depends on the site of application of creams, the occlusive properties of any additional dressing, the percentage of the body surface area covered and total length of use.

Topical tacrolimus has recently been very successfully used to treat atopic dermatitis.[86] This compound inhibits the activation of T cells and, thereby, local cellular infiltration. Phase 3 trials with 0.03% and 0.1% ointments have shown that this form of therapy is both safe efficacious. Even when widely applied, the ointment appears to be well tolerated with no apparent evidence of significant unwanted effects such as infections. The related compound pimecrolimus has a similar mode of action.

Removal of non-specific and allergenic triggers

An important aspect of management is to remove both specific and non-specific triggers. These may include soaps, detergents, chemicals, smoke, abrasive clothing, astringents in lotions and various other cosmetics. In general, patients should avoid extremes of temperature and humidity. Excessive sweating tends to exacerbate the disease. Allergy to food and aeroallergens should be determined from the clinical history and also skin prick testing or RAST as necessary. As mentioned above, negative skin prick tests are of high predictive value, whereas positive tests are less so. Infants and young children who are clinically allergic to milk should substitute cow's milk with hydrolysed proteins or more elemental formulas. Although children may be sensitized to a variety of foods, most do not need to avoid more than two or three foods. Furthermore, food allergens become a much less significant trigger after the age of 5, since by this age children have outgrown most of their food allergies. Patients who are sensitized to house dust mite will probably benefit from avoidance measures, although these have to be strictly applied. It is probably sensible to advise patients with eczema not to allow direct skin contact with any allergen to which they are known to be sensitized, such as cat dander or grass pollen, in so far as this is possible. Allergen immunotherapy has not been shown to be beneficial for atopic dermatitis.

There is increasing recognition that allergy to dermatophyte fungi such as *Trichophyton rubrum* and *Malassezia furfur* may play a role in exacerbation of atopic dermatitis. If such organisms are isolated, a course of topical or systemic antifungal therapy may be indicated.

Because of the role of *Staphylococcal* infection in atopic dermatitis, it is often beneficial to manage disease exacerbations with antistaphylococcal antibiotics. The macrolides (including erythromycin, azithromycin or clarithromycin) are usually suitable, although for resistant organisms a penicillinase-resistant penicillin such as flucloxacillin, may be used. Chronic herpes simplex infection may provoke recurrent, severe dermatitis which may be misdiagnosed as bacterial super infection. Punched-out erosions, vesicles and a poor response to antibiotics suggest superadded herpes infection. In patients who are known to have herpes infection, it is advisable to discontinue topical steroid therapy at least temporarily.

Food allergy

Aetiology

True food allergy is IgE-mediated and reflects inappropriate production of IgE against protein allergens in various foodstuffs. Although any food protein may potentially become allergenic, the commonest culprits are: [87]

- Dairy products (milk, cheese, egg), especially in children
- Seafood (fish, prawn, lobster, mussel, etc.)
- Grains (wheat, barley, oats)
- Nuts (ground nuts or peanuts, and tree nuts)
- Soya
- Increasingly, fruit and vegetables.

The European Academy of Allergy and Clinical Immunology (EAACI) has proposed that the term "adverse food reaction" should embrace toxic, non-toxic and immune reactions to foodstuffs (see Table 13). Toxic reactions may occur in anybody who ingests a specific type of food in sufficient quantity, or may result from contamination of food with bacteria or their products. Sometimes, these reactions may resemble allergic reactions: for example, scromboid food poisoning is caused by the ingestion of histamine released by fish such as tuna as a reaction to bacterial spoilage.

Non-toxic food reactions are seen only in certain individuals, and may reflect intolerance of certain foods caused by gut enzyme deficiencies, such as lactose intolerance. This category also includes a wide variety of mixed reactions of unknown mechanism – some of which may be psychosomatic – which encompasses the general observation that some foods do not "agree" with certain people. Many such symptoms are unjustifiably attributed to foods.[88] The best understood and recognised reactions

Table 13. Adverse reactions to foods *

Toxic
- Food poisoning (e.g. scromboid fish poisoning), gastroenteritis, reactions to caffeine or alcohol

Non-toxic
- Intolerance (for example lactose intolerance)
- Miscellaneous reactions of unknown mechanism, some psychosomatic

Immune
- IgE-mediated
  - Immediate (gastrointestinal, respiratory tract, cutaneous, anaphylactic)
  - Immediate and delayed (cutaneous, gastrointestinal)
- Non-IgE-mediated
  - Coeliac disease (gluten sensitive enteropathy)
  - Other food protein-induced gastrointestinal disease (allergic oesophagitis, gastroenteritis, proctocolitis)
  - Heiner's syndrome (food-induced pulmonary haemosiderosis).

*After Bruijnzeel-Koomen C, Ortolani C, Aas K et al.
Adverse reactions to food (EAACI position paper).
Allergy 1995; **50**: 623–635

are those that occur immediately (within 1 hour) of ingestion. IgE-mediated, Type I hypersensitivity responses underlie many such reactions. In addition, there are well-characterized, reproducible late reactions to food proteins not mediated by IgE, which include gluten-sensitive enteropathy (coeliac disease) and other forms of food protein-induced enteropathy (see further).

Prevalence and natural history

Conventional wisdom suggests that food allergies are most commonly acquired in the first year of life, with a peak prevalence of 6–8% at 1 year of age, which falls during late childhood and then plateaus at about 1–2% of the population through adulthood.[89-91] It is clear that milk and peanut allergy alone now account for a greater prevalence than this.[92, 93] The well known longitudinal study cohort of all children born on the Isle of Wight in 1989[94] showed that, by the age of 4, 0.5% had suffered an allergic reaction to peanut. 4 years later, 1.6% had suffered such a reaction, and twice as many showed positive peanut skin prick tests.

This represents a trebling of the prevalence in just 4 years.[95] In Avon, UK, the Avon Longitudinal Study of Parents and Children (ALSPAC) produced similar findings.[96] In the USA, where peanut consumption is much higher, over 7% of adults and children are now sensitized.[97]

Food allergies, particularly to milk, egg and grains, are most commonly acquired in the first years of life, which corresponds to the time at which these foods were introduced into the infants' diet. They may, however, appear at any age. Milk and egg allergy are commonly outgrown. 85% of children with milk allergy will be able to tolerate milk by the age of 3.[98] Peanut, tree nut, fish and shellfish allergy are much more likely to persist. For example, one study[99] showed that 75% of peanut allergic patients followed for 10 years continued to have reactions to accidental peanut exposure.

Clinical features of IgE-mediated adverse food reactions

These range in severity from mild to severe, including anaphylaxis. They are summarized in Table 14. Onset is soon after ingestion of the food, usually within 10 minutes, and nearly always within 30 minutes.

Oral allergy syndrome

This is seen more often in adults than children. Immediate itching and swelling of the throat, tongue and lips occurs, often after the ingestion of certain fruits, nuts or vegetables. This sometimes develops *de novo*, but more often arises from

Table 14. Symptoms of IgE-mediated food allergy

Oral allergy syndrome
Urticaria/angioedema
Exacerbations of atopic dermatitis
Immediate gastrointestinal symptoms (vomiting, colic, diarrhoea)
Respiratory symptoms (cough, wheeze, rhinorrhoea, laryngospasm, asphyxia, respiratory arrest)
Anaphylaxis

cross-reactivity of allergens in fruits and vegetables with allergens of a similar structure in pollens and latex (used in packaging). Three of the best known associations are:

- Birch pollen oral allergy syndrome: patients with birch pollen hayfever develop oral allergy symptoms with related allergens in fruits of the *Rosaceae* family (any fruit with a pip or stone, as well as hazelnuts and carrots)
- Mugwort oral allergy syndrome: patients with weed pollen hayfever develop symptoms with celery or carrots
- Latex oral allergy syndrome: patients sensitized to latex proteins develop oral allergy syndrome with banana, kiwi fruit, avocado, sweet chestnut, sweet pepper, tomato and potato.

Since cooking often denatures fruit and vegetable allergens, cooked or processed fruits are very much less likely to cause reactions.

Urticaria/angioedema

This may be localized (round the face and mouth) or generalized. Again, the acute and reproducible onset after eating the culprit food is usually obvious. It should be noted that most patients with urticaria/angioedema have "idiopathic" disease in which food allergy plays no role. In these patients, there is no history of symptoms being immediately and reproducibly triggered by exposure to a particular food.

Gastrointestinal symptoms

These include immediate nausea, vomiting and abdominal pain. Diarrhoea may occur 1–2 hours later. Reactions may be explosive and impressive, as may be the speed of recovery when the patient vomits back the food.

Respiratory symptoms

These include laryngeal oedema (a feeling of closing up of the throat causing hoarseness) and wheeze. This may progress rapidly to asphyxia and respiratory arrest, with secondary hypotension.[100] This is often seen in tandem with gastrointestinal symptoms.

Severe and fatal reactions
Food allergy is a major cause of fatal allergic reactions[101] and is the commonest cause of childhood anaphylaxis in the UK.[102] Symptoms may include severe gastrointestinal and respiratory manifestations with hypotension, causing dizziness and syncope (in infants this may be manifest as clumsiness, sleepiness and inattention).

Exacerbation of other atopic diseases
Food allergies are more common in atopic children and should always be suspected in children with asthma, allergic rhinitis and atopic dermatitis. Food allergies are well-documented causes of exacerbations of rhinitis, atopic dermatitis[103] and asthma[104] in children, and so proper management of these diseases includes investigation and treatment of possible food allergy. Food allergies seem to play a less prominent role in the regulation of day-to-day severity of asthma and atopic dermatitis in adults. Nevertheless, all asthmatics are at greater risk of severe bronchospasm from food allergic reactions, and so such reactions should always be carefully identified.

Peanut and tree nut allergy
Peanuts are not actually "nuts": they grow in shells under the ground and are more related to legumes (peas, beans and lentils). Nevertheless "tree" nut (hazelnut, pistachio, almond, brazil, walnut, cashew) and peanut allergy commonly co-exist. Peanut allergy develops in young children who almost always have one or more other atopic diseases (eczema, asthma, allergic rhinitis and other food allergies). The median age of onset is 2 years. There is increased incidence of peanut allergy (7%) in siblings.[105] Tree nut allergy develops later in childhood. Nut allergies often persist into adulthood, although symptoms remit in a minority of patients.

Although peanut allergy is a major cause of severe reactions, the clinical spectrum of reactions varies widely. "Worst ever" reactions range from mild urticaria (50%) through asthma and/or laryngeal oedema (35%–40%), while 10% have life-threatening dyspnoea and/or hypotension.[106]

Cow's milk and egg allergy

Cow's milk and egg allergy usually develop in the first year of life, corresponding to the introduction into the diet of these foodstuffs. Again, children typically have severe atopic diseases such as eczema and/or asthma. Reactions are usually mild but can be severe. 50–70% of milk allergic children have cutaneous symptoms, 50–60% gastrointestinal symptoms and 20–30% respiratory symptoms. A small number of exclusively breast-fed infants may react to cow's milk protein in the mother's milk. The commonest gastrointestinal symptoms are colic, vomiting and diarrhoea. As recounted above, these allergies are frequently outgrown (90% of children by the age of 5).

Clinical diagnosis

History

As with all atopic diseases, correct diagnosis depends on a very careful history supported by skin prick tests and, sometimes, challenge tests. The purpose of the history is to establish a clear and reproducible relationship between exposure to a foodstuff and the onset of a suggestive symptom. If the patient does not already suspect such a relationship, then progress is likely to be limited. If such a relationship is suspected, the history should be amplified to include:

- A full description of the symptoms and signs
- The timing from ingestion of food to onset of symptoms
- The frequency with which reactions have occurred
- The approximate quantity of food required to evoke a reaction.

Often this process is straightforward, for example with a

patient who experiences lip-swelling and urticaria every time he/she eats shellfish. Children also tend to be straightforward in giving a history and do not generally believe that they have food allergy unless they had reactions that made them feel ill. At the other end of the spectrum are patients who produce long lists of vague symptoms with little clear temporal relationship to the ingestion of particular foodstuffs, and who believe that the allergist can produce for them a list of foods to avoid which will change their lives. Such expectations are wholly unrealistic. Adults, as well as anxious parents, frequently place themselves or their children on very restricted and potentially nutritionally inadequate diets because of vague, ill-founded beliefs, including beliefs that such diets will modify children's behaviour.

Sinister symptoms not directly attributable to allergy (abdominal pain, loss of weight or appetite, change of bowel habit, blood or mucus in stools, rectal bleeding, failure to thrive in infants) should be investigated in their own right, usually by a gastroenterologist.

Examination
This should be directed towards other manifestations of atopic disease (rhinitis, eczema, asthma, urticaria) as well as thorough abdominal examination. Related atopic diseases must be evaluated and managed in their own right.

Food Diaries
Food diaries are sometimes, but not always, helpful. They may be useful in highlighting the persistence of symptoms when an incorrectly identified "suspect" food is eliminated but allergic symptoms persist, or in identifying obscure allergens not immediately apparent to the patient.

Clinical and laboratory testing
Skin prick testing
Skin prick tests for common food allergens have a negative predictive value of > 95%. Thus, a properly performed and

valid negative skin prick test essentially excludes IgE-mediated food hypersensitivity. The converse is not true, however, since many patients have positive skin prick tests to food allergens in the absence of any clinical sequelae: the positive predictive value of skin prick tests for clinically significant food allergy is < 50%. Nevertheless, any severe reaction reproducibly associated with a particular food in the presence of a positive skin prick test is considered diagnostic. In cases where reproducible, allergic sounding reactions to suspected foods are not confirmed by skin prick testing, a diagnostic challenge must be performed (see later).

It is vital to note that many commercial allergen extracts for skin prick testing frequently lack labile proteins responsible for reactions to many fruits and vegetables. In such cases it is better to perform "prick prick" testing with the suspect foodstuffs, that is pricking the food to be tested and then the skin of the patient. This may also be used for other substances when commercial skin prick test extracts are not available, for example with spices.

RAST

RAST is useful in patients who cannot stop antihistamines, those using topical or systemic steroids, or those with dermographism or widespread skin disease such as eczema. Again, a good history combined with a positive RAST is considered diagnostic. It is possible to quantify standardized, commercial RAST such as CAP RAST® to increase the positive predictive accuracy for egg, milk and fish allergies (Table 15).[107] Patients above these thresholds may be considered reactive. Patients below these thresholds may or may not be reactive, and this should be investigated by challenge. These tests are also useful in suggesting when patients may lose clinical reactivity on follow-up (that is, they "outgrow" their food allergy), but this is usually verified by challenge.

RAST testing to panels of food allergens is available privately and commercially. Because of the low positive predictive value of such tests, they may produce many

Table 15. 95% positive predictive values for clinical reactions to foods using the CAP–RAST system*

Foodstuff	Serum specific IgE concentration (kU/L)	Follow-up threshold†
Egg (> 2 years old)	≥ 7.0	≤ 1.5
Egg (≤ 2 years old)	≥ 2.0	
Milk (≤ 2 years old)	≥ 5.0	≤ 7.0
Peanut	≥ 14.0	≤ 5.0
Fish	≥ 20.0	
Tree nuts	≥ 15.0	

*From Sampson HA. Utility of food-specific IgE concentrations in predicting symptomatic food allergy. *J Allergy Clin Immunol* 2001; **170**: 891–896.
†Thresholds at which food reactions are no longer likely when patients are followed up.

positive reactions of no clinical relevance, thus compounding patient anxiety. In general they should be avoided.

Food Challenges
Open food challenge
This is very useful, especially for demonstrating lack of food reactivity to patients when such reactivity is considered unlikely. It is also useful in cases where patients have positive skin prick tests to foodstuffs to which they have never been exposed, and where the possibility of a reaction cannot be predicted or ruled out.

Single-blind challenge
This is also very useful in daily clinical allergy practice, confirming or refuting possible food allergy reactions. The food must be concealed in a suitable vehicle, such as capsules, milkshakes, puddings, soup, mashed potatoes, hamburgers or fruit juice. Dried food extracts with which to "spike" the vehicle foods are ideal for this purpose.

Double-blind, placebo-controlled food challenge
This is the gold standard test if organized properly. Protocols vary, but the essential point is that neither the clinician nor the patient is aware of the order of challenge.

The timing between successive challenges must be long enough to allow suspected symptoms to develop: this may necessitate evaluation over several days. Negative challenge must be confirmed by observation of the patient eating the food in normal form and quantity without any problems.

These procedures are not without some risk and must be performed by an experienced allergist in hospital where resuscitation facilities are immediately available, particularly in a case of suspected severe reactions. Informed consent must be obtained from patients or parents.

Management

This must be directed at a strategy to remove or eliminate reactions caused by food allergy. Conversely, since it is clear that food allergies may contribute to the clinical features of asthma and atopic dermatitis, particularly in children, a thorough evaluation of these diseases is not complete without consideration of possible food allergies and management where appropriate.

The principles of management of food allergy are listed in Table 16. In food allergy of any degree, avoidance of the causative food or foods is the cornerstone of management. In the case of mild reactions, such as oral allergy syndrome or mild food-induced urticaria, patients often learn by experience, after suitable education as to the range and nature of the problem, which foods to avoid. With such mild reactions, it is often sufficient for the patient to carry a supply of a fast-acting, non-sedating anti-histamine such as acrivastine for use intermittently in the event of

Table 16. Principles of management of food allergy
• Avoidance
• Education, usually by an allergy dietician
• Reassessment and reiteration
• Anti-histamines
• Auto-injector adrenaline pens
• Written management plan
• Local school surveillance
• Liaison with, and support from, professional and lay societies

accidental exposure. With more serious reactions, patient education is key. In infants allergic to milk, advice about suitable replacement formulae, usually milk hydrolysates, must be provided. Avoidance of products such as milk and eggs can be a daunting task for many parents. Thus, education and provision of information is essential. This may be obtained nowadays not only from health professionals, but also from interested Societies (see Appendix 2). Food manufacturers are becoming increasing "allergy aware" in providing milk, egg and nut-free products. The other side of this coin is that many food manufacturers declare that products "may contain a trace of" a particular foodstuff just to be on the safe side. It is for this reason that patients must acquire the skills of practical avoidance. These must be provided by an allergy dietician. An important parallel role of the dietician is to ensure that elimination diets are nutritionally adequate. Dicticians can also provide recipes and moral support.

Reassessment of patients is necessary to reinforce advice about food avoidance and treatment, particularly with the correct usage of adrenaline auto-injector pens, and to consider the possibility that patients may have lost or "outgrown" their food allergy.

Patients with severe food allergic reactions must be provided with written action plans,[106] which usually specify the rapid use of a fast-acting, non-sedating anti-histamine for mild reactions or auto-injector adrenaline pens for severe reactions. The diagnosis of severe food allergy creates alarm in parents and GPs. Having gone through a phase of under-management, there is now a tendency for GPs to prescribe auto-injector adrenaline pens for all patients. This is inappropriate. It is difficult for the non-specialist to manage these patients, and they should be seen in major allergy centres. The nature of the symptoms and the subsequent action to be taken must be clearly explained to patients or their parents. Furthermore, these plans must be transmitted to works or school medical personnel. In the case of school children, the local

Paediatric Community Physician is responsible for school care and should be informed, with parental consent, of the address of the child's school and the written treatment plan provided. All patients with severe reactions should have two adrenaline pens both at home and at work/school, and should carry one pen with them at all times, especially when visiting "unknown territories" such as unfamiliar restaurants.

Non-IgE-mediated adverse food reactions

Enterocolitis, proctocolitis and enteropathy

Dietary protein proctocolitis

This is a cause of blood and mucus appearing in the stools of otherwise well-looking infants. It is caused by a non-IgE-mediated immune response directed most commonly at cow's milk protein. The mean age at diagnosis is 60 days. In breast-fed infants the cow's milk is transmitted in the mother's breast milk. Similar reactions may occur in response to soya formulae. The disease is not more common in children at risk of atopy.

Dietary protein enteropathy and enterocolitis

These are characterized by protracted diarrhoea, vomiting, malabsorption and failure to thrive, and sometimes bloating, oedema, and hypoalbuminaemia. Symptoms usually begin in the first few months of life. Reaction to cow's milk principally, but also soya, egg, cereals and seafood have been implicated. They sometimes follow viral gastroenteritis. Reactions probably involve food protein-specific T cells, but not IgE.

The differential diagnosis of these conditions is wide but includes IgE-mediated food allergy and lactose intolerance. The diagnosis is based on improvement of symptoms following elimination diets and relapse following re-exposure. In general, a paediatric gastroenterologist should manage them. They commonly resolve within 1–2 years.

Coeliac disease

Also known as gluten-sensitive enteropathy, this disease is a T cell-mediated reaction against wheat gluten or related rye and barley proteins and causes inflammatory infiltration of the intestinal mucosa. It often occurs in infants after weaning onto cereals. Exclusion of gluten from the diet results in amelioration. Symptoms reflect malabsorption, with failure to thrive, anaemia and wasting. Additional symptoms are varied and may include diarrhoea, abdominal pain, vomiting, bone pain and aphthous ulcers. Subclinical or minimal disease may delay diagnosis into adulthood. A related disease is dermatitis herpetiformis, a gluten-responsive dermatitis characterized by pruritic, erythematous papules and/or vesicles distributed symmetrically on the extensor surfaces of the elbows and knees and sometimes on the face, buttocks, neck and trunk.

Testing for IgM anti-endomysial and anti-gliadin antibodies has facilitated diagnosis of coeliac disease. Detectable antibody is associated with an excellent positive (91–100%) and negative (80–98%) predictive value for diagnosing the disease. The gold standard investigation is, however, duodenal biopsy, which is usually warranted when the disease is strongly suspected. If the symptoms are not compelling, a negative endomysial antibody test is usually taken as sufficient evidence of absence of the disease.

Lactose intolerance

Lactose constitutes the majority of the carbohydrate content of human and cow's milk. It is digested by the intestinal enzyme lactase. Congenital lactase deficiency is extremely rare, but acquired deficiency may develop transiently in children as early as 3–5 years of age, particularly children of African or Asian origin. Lactase deficiency is often temporary and may occur in response to malnutrition or following gastrointestinal infections. Lactase deficiency causes bloating, colic and diarrhoea after ingesting dairy products, although features of acute

IgE-mediated allergy are absent. The diagnosis is made by oral lactose challenge tests or hydrogen breath test. Strict milk avoidance is not always necessary, and the prognosis in the case of transient lactase deficiency is generally good.

Irritable bowel syndrome

At present, there is no firm evidence that adverse reactions to foods play a role in the pathogenesis of irritable bowel syndrome. Nevertheless, exclusion of a range of foodstuffs (most commonly milk, wheat and eggs) has been claimed to relieve symptoms in a subset of patients.[108] Other physical bowel disorders must be excluded, and the disease is best managed by a gastroenterologist.

Migraine and epilepsy

The relationship of foods to central nervous system disorders has been the subject of much controversy. At present, there is no firm evidence that food allergy plays a role in the pathogenesis of these diseases. Some foods have been said to provoke migraine because of their chemical content (for example, tyramine in cheese and chocolate). A few studies[109] have suggested that elimination diets may ameliorate these diseases, but further studies are necessary. Management lies within the realm of interested neurologists in consultation with dieticians.

Drug allergy

The spectrum of adverse reactions to drugs

The spectrum of clinical adverse reactions to drugs is summarized in Table 17. Symptoms caused by overdosage, unwanted effects and drug interactions may be observed and predicted in any patient. Unpredictable or idiosyncratic reactions may result from intolerance, congenital metabolic deficiency or immune reactions. Some drugs may cause direct mast cell degranulation with histamine release in susceptible individuals in the absence of an immunological response: clinically these reactions resemble IgE-mediated drug allergy.

Table 17. Spectrum of adverse reactions to drugs

Reactions that may occur in any patient
- Overdosage
  - Toxic reactions to drugs caused by excessive dosages and/or impaired secretion
- Unwanted effect
  - Undesirable effect of a drug at recommended dosage
- Drug interaction
  - Influence of one drug on the efficacy or toxicity of another drug

Reactions occurring only in susceptible individuals
- Drug intolerance
  - A low threshold for the therapeutic or unwanted effects of a drug
- Drug idiosyncracy
  - Genetically determined abnormal reaction to a drug caused by metabolic or enzyme deficiency (e.g. reactions in glucose-6-phosphate dehydrogenase deficiency, porphyria, alcohol sensitivity)
- Drug allergy
  - Immunologically mediated hypersensitivity reaction to a drug, or one or more metabolites, or a complex of the drug with endogenous body protein
- Drug pseudo-allergy
  - Reaction with the same clinical manifestations as a Type I IgE-mediated allergic reaction, but caused by a non-specific effect on mast cells causing direct histamine release. Aspirin-sensitivity may be partly explained by this mechanism.

Immunological reactions to drugs

Drug allergy is defined as an adverse reaction to a drug caused by a specific immune response either directly to the drug or one or more of its metabolites alone, or to a drug bound to a body protein such as albumin. Such binding alters the structure of the drug/protein complex, rendering it antigenic. Hypersensitivity reactions to drugs or drug/protein complexes embrace all four of the classical "hypersensitivity" reactions originally described by Coombs and Gell (Table 18). Immediate immunological reactions to drugs, which typically cause urticarial rashes and systemic features of anaphylaxis such as bronchospasm, urticaria and hypotension, are usually IgE-mediated (Type I hypersensitivity). More delayed reactions may be mediated by antibody-dependent cytolysis, immune complexes or T cell-mediated immunity. These reactions typically involve the skin, causing rashes which may be very severe, or disorders of the peripheral blood, kidney or liver. Some drugs, such as penicillin, have been implicated in causing all of these types of allergic reaction. In many cases, the precise mechanisms underlying the reactions to drugs are poorly defined.

Table 18. Types of hypersensitivity reactions caused by drugs		
Type I	Immediate, IgE-mediated	Anaphylaxis, urticaria/angioedema, bronchospasm, hypotension
Type II	IgG and IgM-dependent complement-mediated cytolysis	Leucopaenia, vasculitis, rashes, interstitial nephritis
Type III	Immune complexes with IgG and IgM	Serum sickness, vasculitis, rashes, fever
Type IV	T cell-mediated reactions	Contact sensivity, delayed rashes

A precise estimate of the prevalence of drug allergy is virtually impossible to ascertain because reactions are under-reported, there is often difficulty in establishing a clear diagnosis and there are few well-developed diagnostic tests or centres with experience in their use.

Allergy to penicillin and other beta-lactam antibiotics

Penicillins may induce an IgE response, with consequent risk of acute urticaria/angioedema, bronchospasm or anaphylaxis on further exposure. They may also induce delayed, T cell-mediated hypersensitivity which typically causes skin rashes which may be severe (Figure 11). Cephalosporins and monobactams may cause similar reactions, but less frequently. Because patterns of antibiotic usage change with time and local medical practices,[110] the patterns of drugs likely to cause allergy change too, and is important to monitor such changes by pharmacosurveillance.[111]

Allergic reactions during anaesthesia

Anaphylaxis during general anaesthesia is an increasingly important problem for the general practitioner, anaesthetist and allergist. Systematic investigation requires expertise

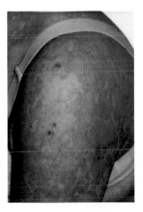

Figure 11. Urticaria caused by allergy to penicillin, showing a wheal and flare response. Reproduced with permission from Holgate ST, Church MK, Lichtenstein LM. *Allergy. Second Edition*. London: Mosby. 2001. (Courtesy of Professor P Friedman)

and should be performed in a specialist allergy centre. It is, however, the responsibility of the medical practitioner (usually an anaesthetist or dentist) "causing" the reaction to document clinical signs and symptoms on the anaesthetic chart, with clear documentation of the times of administration of anaesthetic drugs, as well as any treatment administered, in relationship to the temporal progression of signs and symptoms. Clear recommendations for this procedure have been published by the Association of Anaesthetists of Great Britain and Ireland and the British Society for Allergy and Clinical Immunology[112] (also available at the web site www.aagbi.org).

IgE-medicated reactions to drugs used to induce paralysis during anaesthesia (neuromuscular blocking drugs such as suxamethonium and atracurium) are a rare but serious cause of anaphylaxis during general anaesthesia. The aminosteroids (such as rocuronium and vecuronium) are also an increasingly frequent cause of anaphylaxis. Atracurium and mivacurium may also act directly on mast cells in the absence of an immunological reaction to cause histamine release. Opiate analgesics may also do this.[112]

Latex allergy is an increasingly frequent cause of perioperative anaphylaxis (see *Latex allergy*). The administration of rectal nonsteroidal anti-inflammatory drugs for post-operative analgesia may cause bronchospasm and urticaria in aspirin-sensitive patients (see further).

Local anaesthetics, typically administered for dental procedures, are commonly suspected to have caused immediate allergic reactions. In fact, true allergy to drugs such as lignocaine is extremely rare. Symptoms are much more commonly caused by anxiety (fainting), overdosage or intolerance (a low threshold for unwanted effects). Occasionally, reactions may be seen to preservatives or to latex in dental anaesthetic cartridges or dental dams. Nevertheless, it is essential to establish an accurate diagnosis: the only alternative is for the patient never to have another local anaesthetic. Skin prick tests for lignocaine allergy are not validated, so the diagnosis can only be established by challenge in a specialist allergy centre or department of oral medicine.

Other drugs

Many other drugs, including anticonvulsants, antibiotics, antihypertensive agents and even herbal remedies may cause delayed skin rashes (Figure 12), which may occasionally progress to bullous eruptions and even life-threatening exfoliative dermatitis. The mechanisms are unclear but likely involve T cell-mediated hypersensitivity. Such reactions are often associated with renal or hepatic derangement or leucopaenia. Similarly, many drugs rarely cause urticaria/angioedema: the mechanisms involved in these isolated cases are often ill defined.

Allergic reactions to vaccines

Although formation of IgE antibodies to vaccines such as tetanus and diphtheria toxids is well documented,[113] allergic reactions occurring after re-injection are extremely rare. A similar situation pertains with insulin, where up to 40% of diabetics treated with heterologous (bovine or porcine) insulin develop IgE antibodies, but clinical hypersensitivity reactions are extremely uncommon.[114]

Sensitivity reactions can occur when egg-allergic patients are vaccinated with vaccines containing egg protein. These vaccines include yellow fever, mumps, rabies, influenza and rubella. Again, significant clinical reactions are extremely

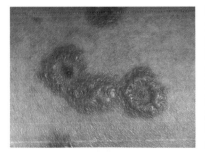

Figure 12. Erythema multiforme induced by an anticonvulsant. Reproduced with permission from Holgate ST, Church MK, Lichtenstein LM. *Allergy. Second Edition.* London: Mosby. 2001. (Courtesy of Professor P Friedman)

rare. For example, severe anaphylactic reactions to influenza vaccination have been reported to occur at a rate of 0.024 per 100,000 vaccinations.[115] Egg-sensitive individuals should not receive such vaccinations unless the need is great, in which case a negative skin prick test to the vaccine provides considerable reassurance that anaphylaxis will not occur. If a patient does suffer a severe anaphylactic reaction to a vaccine, further vaccination with the same vaccine is contraindicated.

Aspirin and nonsteroidal anti-inflammatory drugs

Some patients develop acute reactions to ingestion of aspirin or related nonsteroidal anti-inflammatory drugs (such as ibuprofen, indomethacin, etc.). The spectrum of clinical symptoms includes respiratory tract symptoms (acute rhinitis, bronchospasm), urticaria/angioedema and gastrointestinal symptoms (nausea, vomiting, diarrhoea).

These reactions do not represent a true immunological reaction to these drugs, but rather reflect acute release of leukotrienes in the affected target organs. Direct degranulation of mast cells by aspirin may be a contributory factor. A common feature of all responsible drugs is that they inhibit the enzyme cyclo-oxygenase 1 (COX-1), which produces prostaglandins such as PGE_2 which are thought to be necessary to protect against excessive leukotriene release in susceptible individuals. Since an immunological reaction is not involved, diagnosis must be made by direct challenge (usually in a specialist allergy centre). A small proportion of aspirin-sensitive patients have similar symptoms with high dosages of paracetamol. The reason for this is unexplained. There is increasing evidence that the newer NSAIDs celecoxib, rofecoxib and etoricoxib, which inhibit the alternative isoform of cyclo-oxgenase (COX-2), are tolerated by the majority of aspirin-sensitive patients, although it must be remembered that these drugs do not substitute for the antiplatelet effects of aspirin. Angiotensin-converting enzyme (ACE) inhibitors, commonly used for the treatment of hypertension and cardiac failure, can also cause angioedema. This is probably because ACE also breaks down vasoactive kinins released locally in the skin, increasing local vascular permeability.

Diagnosis

As with all allergy diagnosis, the single most important facet is an accurate detailed history which clearly links administration of a drug with the development of symptoms. In the case of perioperative anaphylaxis, a complete anaesthetic record must be obtained (see earlier). For other reactions, a detailed record of symptoms and their temporal relationship to the ingestion or injection of drugs is essential. Enquiries must be made about *every* drug taken at the time of the reaction, including "non-formulary" drugs such as herbal remedies. True drug allergy implies prior exposure to the offending drug, or a cross-reactive drug, and so a detailed past drug history is appropriate. IgE-mediated reactions to drugs typically occur within seconds if the drug is injected, or minutes if it is swallowed (unless the preparation is enteric-coated). Non-IgE-mediated reactions occur later (hours or days). In many patients labelled as being "allergic" to antibiotics such as penicillin, a clear history of symptoms suggestive of an IgE-mediated reaction (bronchospasm, hypotension, urticaria/angioedema within minutes of drug ingestion) is lacking: most often the history is of a rash, or other signs or symptoms, appearing at a variable period after administration of the drug for an unspecified acute febrile illness. Such patients are unlikely to have IgE-mediated penicillin allergy.

One of the most important aspects of drug allergy diagnosis is to identify or exclude IgE-mediated allergic reactions that may potentially cause rapid and life-threatening anaphylaxis. More delayed reactions are less likely to be life-threatening, and the simple expedient of stopping the drug is treatment enough.

Skin prick testing

A positive skin prick test to a drug implies acute, local histamine release caused by an IgE-mediated hypersensitivity reaction to the drug or a direct action of the drug on mast cells. Skin prick tests cannot predict more delayed, non-IgE-mediated reactions to drugs such as rashes. Presently, there is no available test that can predict such delayed reactions.

The major and minor "allergens" of penicillin (penicilloyl polylysine [PPL] and minor determinant mixture [MDM]) are commercially available for skin prick testing. Many allergists, when testing for penicillin allergy, also include ampicillin and amoxicillin, since there is increasing evidence that some patients may become sensitized to unique determinants in these penicillins, while having negative skin prick tests to the penicillin major and minor determinants. As with all skin prick tests for allergy, these have good negative predictive value, reassuring the physician and the patient that an anaphylactic reaction is unlikely, but poor positive predictive value, since false positive reactions do occur. Nevertheless, a good history of symptoms of histamine release occurring soon after the administration of a drug, coupled with a positive skin prick test, is usually regarded as diagnostic of IgE-mediated allergy to the drug. If not commercially available, it is often possible to perform skin prick tests directly with prescribable solutions of drugs, such as solutions of antibiotics for intravenous use, injectable anaesthetic drugs or dissolved tablets. Drugs amenable to skin prick testing in this way are listed in Table 19. Again, a negative test implying the absence of an IgE-mediated response to the drug is reassuring, but these "ad hoc" tests have yet to be systematically validated in terms of their predictive value. It is sometimes appropriate to proceed to intradermal testing with antibiotics if skin prick tests are negative. This involves injecting greater quantities of drug in small volumes under the skin and inspecting for an acute wheal, and adds to the predictive value of the testing.

Table 19. Drugs suitable for skin prick tests of IgE-mediated allergy
Antibiotics Penicillin Cephalosporins Tetracyclines, macrolides
Anaesthetic drugs Muscle relaxants Intravenous anaesthetics
Enzymes Streptokinase, urokinase
Chemotherapeutic drugs Cis-platinum
Others Insulin Vaccines

Skin prick testing with opiates is unreliable since these drugs often produce non-specific positive tests caused by a direct effect of the drug on local mast cells.[116] Muscle-relaxing drugs such as suxamethonium may have a similar effect in some patients.

Radioallergosorbent tests (RAST)
Commercial tests such as the CAP RAST® are available for a limited number of drug allergens including amoxicilloyl, ampicilloyl, penicilloyl G, penicilloyl B, cefaclor and suxamethonium. These tests are subject to the same limitations as skin prick tests and must be interpreted in the light of the clinical history.

Other tests
In the light of increasing evidence that late drug reactions, especially skin rashes, may be caused by T cell-mediated hypersensitivity reactions to drugs, skin patch tests and tests for T cell activation by drugs[117] are being investigated for the diagnosis of late drug reactions, but their use is still experimental. Similarly, tests for IgE-mediated basophil

activation by drugs in sensitized patients are presently being evaluated as research tools for diagnostic use.[118]

In any acute severe reaction, elevation of serum tryptase within 1 to 2 hours of the reaction supports the diagnosis of acute mast cell degranulation (IgE-mediated or otherwise), and lends support to the suspicion that a drug or other reaction has been caused by anaphylaxis.

Direct challenge tests

These should be undertaken only in specialist allergy centres when investigations have been exhausted and the diagnosis remains in doubt. Challenge tests should be designed to implicate or exonerate a suspected drug, or to investigate the safety of an alternative, related drug. There is a danger of anaphylaxis and attendant staff should be experienced in its management.

Management of drug allergy

Acute anaphylaxis should be treated in its own right (see *Anaphylaxis*). It is essential to withdraw the offending drug immediately, but this may be difficult in patients taking a variety of drugs. Anaesthetic reactions must be fully investigated, especially in patients having had a reaction when further operations are likely to be necessary. In addition to identifying drugs causing reactions, an equally important aspect of management is to identify suitable alternative drugs. These may be suggested by negative skin prick tests backed up in same cases by direct challenge. Such investigations should be undertaken at specialist allergy centres. Patients with severe drug allergies should be encouraged to make this widely known to all medical and dental personnel, and may wish to carry a personal warning such as a medical alert bracelet or pendant. In some cases, such as penicillin allergy or aspirin sensitivity, it may be helpful to provide patients with a complete list of drugs to which they may react.

Latex allergy

Latex and latex allergy

Latex is derived from natural rubber, which is itself composed of various polymers of isoprene. Natural rubber is the 1:4 *cis* polymer. Rubber is collected from the rubber tree *Hevea brasiliensis*, which grows naturally in the Amazon basin but has now been exported to South-East Asia and West Africa. This should not be confused with the domestic "rubber plant" *Ficus elastica*.

The raw rubber can be processed in two basic ways. "Dry" rubber is produced by acid coagulation. It is hard and resilient, and is used to make products such as tyres (see Table 20). Although it contains little protein, this is sometimes enough to be allergenic. Latex concentrate is ammonia/alkali precipitated and is used to make products such as condoms/diaphragms, adhesives, foam, gloves and elastic (Table 20). The latex protein content of such products is much higher. Latex may thus be found in a wide variety of medical devices and household products (Table 21). "Powdered" surgical gloves are lubricated with polysaccharides such as corn starch, which tend to absorb latex protein allergens and create a "mist" of latex-containing particles which, like pollens, may be potent allergens when inhaled.[119] Although synthetic rubber gloves

Table 20. Latex-processing for particular products	
Dry rubber	**Latex concentrate**
Tyres	Gloves
Latex goods	Adhesives
Shoes	Elastic
Engineering	Foam
Cables and tubes	Carpets
Vehicles	Imitation leather
	Contraceptives

Table 21. Products that *may* contain latex	
Medical devices	**Household products**
Urinary catheters	Balloons*
Blood pressure cuffs	Condoms/diaphragms*
Dental dams/blocks*	Elasticated fabrics*
Bulb syringes	Carpet backing, foam underlays
Enema syringes*	Nappies
Intravenous access injection ports	Incontinence pads
Manual resuscitators	Rubber gloves
Pulse oximeters	(washing, gardening)
Penrose surgical drains	Infant pacifiers ("dummies")
Stethoscope tubing	Rubber bands
ET tubes and airways	Rubber bungs, handles,
Tourniquets	shock absorbers
Vascular stockings	Some pencil erasers ("rubbers")
Elastic bandages	Some adhesives
Stretcher mattresses	("rubber solution" glues)

*Reported as sources of allergic sensitization.

(neoprene, nitrile) and condoms (polyurethane) are available, natural rubber gloves are often preferred on grounds of their excellent elasticity and much lower cost.

Latex-sensitized patients produce IgE that recognises one or more proteins present within refined latex, which contains over 200 proteins.[120] Some latex proteins are similar in structure to allergens found in a variety of fruits and vegetables. Thus, some patients sensitized to latex may also become sensitized to these foodstuffs (see further).

Prevalence of latex allergy

Following the original description of latex allergy in 1979, [121] the number of papers on the subject has certainly mushroomed, but it is not clear how far this reflects increased exposure to latex or increasing prevalence of sensitization. The reported incidence of positive RAST tests for latex in unselected populations varies from 1 to 8%, although not all of these patients have clinically significant reactions.[122-126] It has been suggested that healthcare workers using latex gloves are "at risk", but studies addressing this question have produced conflicting results.[127,128] Individual risk may reflect exposure, which is highly variable in hospitals.[129] Patients with congenital urinary dysfunction, who are exposed to multiple surgical procedures as well as catheters, are clearly at risk,[130] although there are no good data to indicate that frequent surgery is a risk factor for latex sensitization in the wider population. Approximately one-third of patients with spina bifida will have a history of reactions to latex products, and should be handled in a "latex-free" environment (see further). Studies on the natural history of latex allergy have revealed no clear temporal sequence for predisposition to latex allergy in atopic subjects, although it certainly affects both children and adults. In general, the prevalence declines with age. At the level of the individual, the risk from occupational exposure is very variable and it has not been possible to define a safe or unsafe degree of exposure.

Clinical manifestations of IgE-mediated Type I hypersensitivity to latex

The principal clinical manifestations of latex Type I hypersensitivity include:

- Urticaria (either locally where contact occurs or generalized)
- Respiratory tract disease (rhinitis, asthma)
- Anaphylaxis (this may be the presenting feature of latex allergy).

The precise constellation of symptoms varies between individuals, but tends to remain fairly constant within an individual, although this may depend on the degree of exposure. As with all IgE-mediated reactions, symptoms are typically immediate (minutes to hours) (Figure 13).

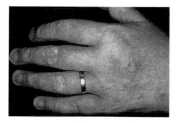

Figure 13. Contact urticaria developing within minutes of wearing latex gloves. Reproduced with permission from Gawkrodger DJ. *Dermatology. Third Edition*. Edinburgh: Churchill Livingstone. 2002.

Diagnosis of latex allergy

Diagnosis can be, but is not usually difficult and, as with all diagnosis of allergic disease, requires a high index of suspicion and a careful clinical history backed up by a positive skin prick test or RAST. While in some patients the diagnosis may be made obvious by rapid development of one or more of the above clinical manifestations developed reproducibly on contact with latex, the disease may present where there is no previous history of latex reactions. Not all patients with severe reactions fall into "high-risk" categories. A further complication is that many household articles may unexpectedly contain latex. Diagnosis therefore requires a careful clinical history which may embrace the patient's occupation, atopic status and the precise circumstances of the clinical reactions. Evidence must be sought of previous similar episodes after contact with rubber articles, particularly household items such as gloves, balloons, and condoms and during dental or surgical procedures. Allergy to fruits containing proteins which cross-react with latex proteins (see further) also supports the diagnosis. A good clinical history has a high sensitivity and specificity for diagnosis of clinical latex allergy.

Clinical suspicion of latex allergy is supported by a positive skin prick test or RAST (Figure 14). As with all skin prick tests for allergy, these tests have a high specificity but poor positive predictive value, since up to 25% of patients with positive skin prick test or RAST have no clinical symptoms.[131] Other approaches to testing include performing

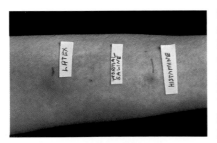

Figure 14. Positive skin prick test to latex. Reproduced with permission from Gawkrodger DJ. *Dermatology. Third Edition.* Edinburgh: Churchill Livingstone. 2002.

skin prick tests with allergenic gloves steeped in saline, skin pricking through suspect articles or wearing, or laying gloves or other suspect articles on a wet hand. Testing should be carried out with resuscitation facilities immediately available, since there is a small risk of anaphylaxis especially in patients having had severe clinical reactions.

In patients where these tests fail to provide evidence of latex-specific IgE when the history is compelling, a direct challenge with latex containing articles may be performed in hospital where suitable resuscitation facilities are available. In some patients, local reactions may reflect not latex allergy but contact hypersensitivity to latex additives (see further). Occasionally, other additives such as casein may cause reactions in milk-allergic patients. For all these reasons, accurate diagnosis is best left to an experienced allergist.

Latex allergy and food allergy

Since some of the major protein allergens found in latex cross-react with similar proteins in fruits, some latex allergic patients may develop allergic reactions to these fruits. Such reactions commonly manifest as an oral allergy syndrome, in which the patient develops localized itching and/or swelling of the tongue and mouth immediately on direct contact with the foodstuff. Occasionally, such reactions may be more severe, causing more generalized urticaria or features of anaphylaxis. Fruits that may cross-react in this way include avocado, banana, tomato, potato, sweet chestnut, sweet pepper and kiwi fruit. It should be remembered that such fruit allergy may also develop independently in the absence of latex allergy. Indeed, such cases are often associated with more severe clinical reactions.

Management of Type I latex hypersensitivity

Key features of the management of latex allergy are summarised in Table 22. The cornerstone of management, as with many allergic reactions, is strict avoidance, since severe reactions, including anaphylactic shock, may occur

Table 22. Management of latex allergy
• Strict avoidance, since anaphylaxis possible
• Written information about the nature of the disease, the dangers, suitable alternatives to rubber, possible reactions to fruits
• Anti-histamines
• Warning bracelet
• Adrenaline pen
• Latex-free environment for procedures
• Non-rubber bungs, vial closures and giving sets

on latex exposure. The patient should be provided with written information about the nature of the disease, the possible dangers, and a list of suitable alternatives to rubber products, particularly gloves and condoms. Such information should be available from an allergy clinic, and is also available from patient lay support groups in the UK, such as the Latex Allergy Support Group and the Anaphylaxis Campaign. All patients should consider wearing a medical alert bracelet or pendant warning that they have latex allergy in case of sudden emergencies requiring surgery. Most patients are advised to carry a supply of fast-acting, non-sedating antihistamine which they might take for less severe reactions, and an auto-injector adrenaline pen for more severe reactions.

With the increasing recognition of latex allergy, many hospitals and dental surgeries are providing a complete latex-free environment for procedures, which includes the use of non-rubber bungs, vial closures and giving sets.[132,133] It is relatively straightforward to substitute latex gloves with substitute vinyl gloves. Particular care must be taken with dental prostheses, such as dams, which may contain latex.

Latex allergy and anaesthesia
Latex should be considered as a possible cause of all episodes of peri-operative anaphylaxis. Although reactions to latex during anaesthesia may be rapid, many are delayed.[134] The manifestations of latex allergy during

anaesthesia typically include hypotension, increased airway pressure and generalized enythema.[135] A French study showed that latex allergy was responsible for 0.5% of all causes of peri-operative anaphylaxis in 1989 but 16.6% of all causes in 1996.[136]

If a reaction does occur, this must be treated and recorded according to the guidelines of the Association of Anaesthetists of Great Britain and Ireland and the BSACI.[135] Patients must be immediately removed from exposure to all items which do or may contain latex. If the item in question is not a well-recognised source of latex exposure, the incident should be reported to the Committee on Safety of Medicines using the "yellow card" reporting system. Strategies for creating a latex-safe surgical environment have been published[137-139] and should be followed for latex-allergic patients.

Latex allergy and dentistry

In many dental practices, routine use is now made of powder-free gloves made of alternative substances such as nitrile. Again, latex allergic reactions during dental procedures may be brought to light by a careful temporal history of the nature the reaction and its proximity to possible latex exposure. Unfortunately, there is as yet no universal databank listing dental devices which may contain latex, but the commonest sources of exposure in dentistry apart from latex gloves are rubber dental dams and local anaesthetic cartridges. Rubber-free alternatives are becoming available. Guidelines for the management of latex allergic dental patients have been published,[140] and should be followed when treating latex-allergic patients.

Patients with suspected latex reactions during anaesthesia and dental procedures should be referred to an allergy clinic for careful evaluation. In general, the onus is on the person "causing" the reaction (i.e. the anaesthetist or the dental surgeon) to provide a careful record of the reaction, along with a temporal sequence of all drugs and prostheses to which the patient was exposed.

Contact sensitivity (Type IV) reactions to latex additives

Quite commonly, local reactions to latex products (such as a rash on the hands after wearing latex gloves) reflect contact hypersensitivity of the patient to latex additives rather than allergy to the latex itself. Latex contains various chemicals which are used as accelerators of vulcanization, such as thiurames, carbamates and benzothiazoles. Contact hypersensitivity to such additives can be readily detected by patch testing performed by an experienced dermatologist. Thiurames may also be found in some cosmetic sponge applicators and horticultural fungicides.

Insect venom allergy

Introduction

Female insects of the order *Hymenoptera* have true stings: honey bees and bumble bees belong to the family of *Apidae*, and hornets and wasps ("yellow jackets" in the USA) to the family of *Vespidae*. The honey bee's stinger is barbed and remains in the skin, whereas the sting of wasps does not. Bee and wasp venoms contain distinctive major protein allergens which have been well characterized. The major allergen of wasp venom is antigen 5, while those of bees include phospholipase A_2 and mellitin. Wasp venom allergens cross-react extensively, whereas those of the honey bee and bumble bee do not.

In Europe, allergy to honey bee sting occurs mainly in bee keepers (those exposed and frequently stung), whereas wasp venom allergy may occur with random, occasional stings.

Natural history of insect venom allergy

Bee or wasp stings may cause allergic reactions, but these are uncommon. Only a minority (1–3%) cause allergic reactions, which may vary widely in severity (see further). All age groups may be affected. Each year about two or three fatal anaphylactic reactions to stings are reported in European countries, and up to 10 in the USA.

Venom-specific IgE antibodies can be found in 30–40% of adults in the few months following a sting. Atopic subjects are at increased risk of becoming sensitized, but both atopic and non-atopic subjects have an approximately equal risk of systemic reactions.[141] The placebo wing of the first double-blind study on venom immunotherapy revealed that 40% of untreated patients with systemic reactions to stings do not react to subsequent stings.[142] The incidence of significant further reactions varies widely in reported studies, but the mean value is 45%. Children with cutaneous

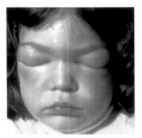

Figure 15. Acute facial swelling following a bee sting, associated with systemic anaphylaxis. Reproduced with permission from Fireman P, Slavin RG. Atlas of Allergies. Second Edition. London: Mosby-Wolfe. 1996.

Table 23. Grading of severity of systemic reactions to insect stings	
Grade 1	Pruritus, urticaria, rhinitis, discomfort
Grade 2	Angioedema, dizziness, abdominal symptoms
Grade 3	Dyspnoea, laryngeal oedema, anxiety
Grade 4	Hypotension, cyanosis, loss of consciousness

systemic reactions are at even lower risk (about 10%) of further systemic reactions, and only at 0.4% risk of further severe reactions.[143] The prognosis is best for those with milder systemic reactions, in children, in those with wasp allergy and when the interval between stings is longer.[144] Thus, contrary to what patients are often told or suspect, for the majority of patients subsequent sting reactions are likely to be less, rather than more, severe. A few patients not reacting to an initial sting may react to a subsequent one.

Clinical features

Local reactions

The "normal" reaction to an insect sting is local pain, oedema and swelling. Some patients experience particularly large local reactions to wasp and bee stings. However large, these are not usually a precursor of systemic reactions.

Systemic reactions. These vary widely in severity from systemic cutaneous reactions to anaphylaxis (Figure 15).[145]

A grading of severity is shown in Table 23. Anaphylactic reactions are typically of rapid onset (within 15 minutes), but may be more delayed. Respiratory symptoms are less common than with allergic reactions to food. A few patients have little or no warning in the way of symptoms before they collapse with hypotension.

Diagnosis

It is important to make the diagnosis of insect venom allergy because of the risk of severe systemic reactions and because allergen immunotherapy is very effective. Diagnosis is based on the history confirmed by skin prick or intradermal testing and measurement of venom-specific IgE in serum by RAST (sensitive tests such as CAP RAST® are now routinely available). Pitfalls include incorrect identification of the stinging insect by the patient and the fact that many patients have positive skin prick tests to both wasp and bee venom yet clinical allergy to only one insect.[146] In fact, clinical sensitivity to both wasp and bee venom simultaneously is extremely uncommon. As with all skin prick tests for allergy, positive venom skin prick tests have a poor positive predictive value for allergic symptoms: up to 25% of adults having no reaction to a further sting will have a positive skin prick test or RAST. RAST are negative in 20% of skin prick test positive subjects,[147] and neither test alone will detect all patients: it is therefore important to do both. Golden[147] has shown that about 30% of patients with a history of systemic reaction to a wasp or bee sting have a negative skin prick test: some 36% of these patients have a positive RAST, but some show negative skin prick test and RAST. If the history is convincing and skin prick testing and RAST are negative, these tests should be repeated in 3–6 months. With such patients, avoidance and preparedness to treat is prudent. When the major allergens of bee and wasp venoms are available in recombinant form, the sensitivity of skin prick testing is likely to increase.[148]

Management

Mild reactions to stings may be treated symptomatically, if necessary, with cold compresses and analgesics, and fast-acting, non-sedating anti-histamines such as acrivastine, loratadine/desloratadine, cetirizine/levocetirizine or fexofenadine taken for a few days. In patients with very extensive local reactions, an additional short course of oral steroids may occasionally be justified.

In patients with systemic reactions, management will be influenced by such factors as:

- The risk of a further reaction
- The natural history of the disease
- The risk of a further sting
- The time interval from the last sting
- The results of skin prick testing and RAST
- The general medical condition of the patient.

All patients with systemic reactions should be given advice on insect avoidance (Table 24) and be provided with emergency medication tailored to fit their symptoms. This should ideally be presented in the form of a written treatment plan. For urticaria, antihistamines and short courses of oral steroids may be provided. For mild asthmatic symptoms, inhaled β_2-agonists can be prescribed for use "as required".

Table 24. Advice on bee and wasp avoidance
• Do not annoy the insects
• Always wear shoes and leg coverings outside
• Avoid highly scented fragrances and cosmetics
• Keep away from flowers when sitting outdoors
• Be careful consuming berries, fruits and sweet drinks outside
• Cover all foods outdoors
• Keep away from places where a lot of food is left open, or the vicinity of litter bins

For severe systemic reactions, medication may include an auto-injector adrenaline pen. Patients should be carefully instructed when and how to use such pens, and this training should be reiterated at intervals. A full description of the management of anaphylaxis is given in *Anaphylaxis.*

Insect venom immunotherapy

Venom immunotherapy is highly effective, protecting about 95% of patients with wasp venom allergy and 80–90% of those allergic to bee venom.[149] Quality of life is also improved.[150] The main disadvantages of immunotherapy are the small but tangible risk of anaphylaxis during treatment, and the time and cost commitments involved. Conventional venom immunotherapy is given with an initial course of incremental injections of pure venom (typically weekly for approximately 10 weeks) followed by maintenance injections given monthly to 3-monthly for a total of 3 years.

The appropriate venom (wasp, honey bee or bumble bee) must be used. Treatment should be administered and monitored at a specialised allergy clinic.

According to British[151] and European[149] guidelines, venom immunotherapy should be offered to all patients with severe and some moderate systemic reactions, particularly those with respiratory and/or cardiovascular symptoms, who have a positive skin prick test and/or RAST to the appropriate venom. This does not include patients with isolated local reactions, however large. Not all patients will meet these criteria at their first presentation (see earlier). Some patients who do meet the criteria may choose not to undergo immunotherapy for reasons of expediency (for example the time required off work and their proximity to an allergy clinic), or because they accept that the natural history of the condition is generally to improve and that their risk of a further sting is low, and will prefer to continue with an emergency treatment plan. Patients at high risk of further stings (such as bee keepers) should be encouraged to undergo immunotherapy, as should elderly patients and those with cardiovascular disease who are more at risk of the effects of anaphylaxis. More severe asthmatics, who are not usually considered suitable for immunotherapy with aeroallergens, may also be considered suitable for venom immunotherapy for this reason. The decision whether or not to undergo immunotherapy should be an informed one made by the patient based on the advice of an experienced allergist. Other groups in which venom immunotherapy is absolutely or relatively contraindicated include:

- Those with other immunological disorders or immunodeficiency
- Patients with malignancy
- Patients treated with β-blockers
- Patients considered unlikely to comply with the therapy regimen
- Pregnancy: immunotherapy is not commenced in pregnancy unless there are exceptional extenuating circumstances, but may usually be continued if a patient becomes pregnant during therapy
- Children: because of the good prognosis of further sting reactions in children, venom immunotherapy is not usually recommended for children.

Although venom immunotherapy is highly effective, a small proportion of patients will have further systemic reactions to insect stings after completing a full course, although these are likely to be milder. At present, it is not possible to identify such patients *a priori*: the loss of a previously positive skin prick test to venom during or after therapy is reassuring, but many fully protected patients continue to have a positive skin prick test. Immunotherapy does not act by abolishing IgE responses, but by shifting T cell allergen responses away from an allergy-promoting Th2-type cytokine profile (see *Definition, pathogenesis and epidemiology*), and inducing the production of anti-allergic cytokines such as IL-10.[152-154] Consequently, the loss of a positive skin prick test during immunotherapy probably reflects the natural history of the disease rather than the protective effects of the immunotherapy itself. The only "acid test" for a "cure" is the demonstration of a lack of systemic response to a further sting in the field. For this reason some patients feel motivated to continue to carry emergency treatment until this occurs.

Anaphylaxis

Anaphylaxis (meaning "against or without protection") refers to the systemic, catastrophic release of mediators from mast cells and basophils. Other mast cell mediators, including leukotrienes, prostaglandins and cytokines are also likely involved.[155] This may be caused by IgE-mediated reactions in allergic patients exposed to agents to which they are sensitized, or by IgE-independent, direct effects of certain agents on mast cells and basophils causing non-immune degranulation. These latter reactions used to be labelled "anaphylactoid", but since both types of reaction have identical sequelae and require identical clinical management, this term has now largely been discontinued.

Aetiology

Recognised causes of anaphylaxis are listed in Table 25. Foods, especially peanuts are common causes of anaphylaxis, and drug allergy, although greatly under

Table 25. Recognized triggers of anaphylaxis
IgE-mediated
Foodstuffs (peanuts, tree nuts, seafood, others)
Drugs (penicillins, anaesthetic agents, others)
Vaccines
Insect venom allergy (*Hymenoptera*)
Latex allergy
Exercise (sometimes in combination with foods or drugs)
IgE-independent
Aspirin and related NSAIDs
ACE inhibitors
Intravenous contrast media
Opioid analgesics
Intravenous anaesthetic drugs
Intravenous immunoglobulins
Plasma expanders
Blood transfusion
Idiopathic

reported, is an increasing cause. The most common foods causing anaphylaxis are peanuts, tree nuts, soya beans, crustaceans, celery, egg, milk, some cereals and white fish such as cod.[156] Almost any food may rarely be implicated. Further information on other allergic triggers of anaphylaxis is provided in other sections. The aetiology of many recurrent cases of anaphylaxis is never revealed (idiopathic anaphylaxis).

Epidemiology

There are few reliable data on the morbidity and mortality of anaphylaxis. This reflects partly the lack of an agreed clinical definition, and partly the fact that anaphylaxis is encountered by such a wide variety of physicians (few of them allergists). A retrospective study of patients presenting to an A&E department in England[157] found that one in 3,500 patients per year develop anaphylaxis in the community. This is likely an underestimation, and furthermore does not include the considerable incidence of anaphylaxis arising in hospital inpatients, which has been assessed at approximately 150 per million subjects hospitalized annually.[158] The number of hospital admissions for anaphylaxis has increased seven-fold in the last decade.[159]

Clinical features

No universally accepted clinical definition of anaphylaxis exists because the syndrome may comprise of a constellation of features, not all of which are seen in every patient. A good working definition is that it involves at least one of two severe features: respiratory distress (which may be due to laryngeal oedema or asthma) and hypotension (which may present as fainting, collapse or loss of consciousness in adults and "floppiness" and inattention in infants and young children). A list of all possible symptoms, with an overall incidence, is shown in Table 26. These symptoms are caused by the effects of histamine, leukotrienes and other mediators on blood vessels and capillaries, smooth muscle, mucus glands and sensory nerve endings.

Table 26. Clinical features of anaphylaxis	
Symptoms	**Overall incidence (%)** [*]
Urticaria/angioedema	88
Laryngeal oedema	56
Dyspnoea, chest tightness	47
Flushing	46
Dizziness, hypotension, fainting	33
Abdominal symptoms (nausea, vomiting, colic, diarrhoea)	30
Rhinitis	16
Headache (especially in exercise-induced anaphylaxis)	15
Itching	5

[*]Different constellations of symptoms occur in different patients according to the aetiological agent.

The clinical picture will vary with the cause. In the case of systemically injected agents (drugs, blood products, insect venom), hypotension and shock predominate. Ingested allergens seem especially to cause lip, facial and laryngeal oedema. Death occurs by suffocation or profound hypotension. The risk of a lethal outcome is greatest in patients with asthma, in the elderly and in patients taking β-blockers or ACE inhibitors, since these drugs hinder the body's adrenergic compensatory mechanisms (as well as the therapeutic actions of administered adrenaline).

Reactions generally begin within 20 minutes of exposure. Prodromal symptoms may also occur and it is important to recognise these symptoms, which include itching and burning of the skin, especially in hair-covered areas of the body, and the feeling of menace or impending doom.

A number of cases of anaphylaxis induced by exercise have been reported. Symptoms typically begin 1–4 hours following prolonged exercise. In some of these patients, anaphylaxis develops only when certain foods (celery, shellfish) or drugs (aspirin and NSAIDs) have also been ingested. In these and other patients, severe symptoms may recur after hours of apparent recovery, so prolonged and close monitoring is essential.

Acute management of anaphylaxis

In any setting where drugs (antibiotics or anaesthetic agents) are administered parenterally, or vaccinations or allergen immunotherapy performed, facilities should be available for the emergency of treatment of anaphylaxis and staff should be trained to recognise the symptoms quickly and respond appropriately.

Recently, consensus guidelines on the emergency treatment of anaphylactic reactions, intended specifically for first medical responders, have been published[160,161] and are summarized in Figures 16 and 17. It should be noted that when a patient carries an adrenaline auto-injector pen because of a perceived danger of severe anaphylaxis, this may be used as an alternative to drawing up 1:1000 adrenaline solution in a syringe. The guidelines have recently been extended[162] to include management of

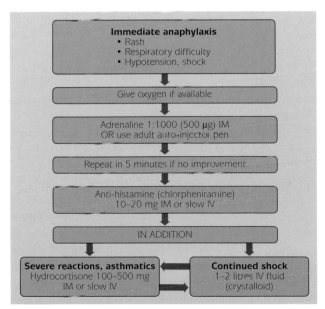

Figure 16. Anaphylactic reactions: treatment of adults by first medical responders.

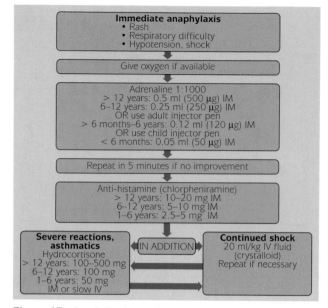

Figure 17. Anaphylactic reactions: treatment for children by first medical responders.

anaphylactic reactions by nurses and other health professionals in the community, who would be likely to have access only to adrenaline. These community guidelines, summarized in Figures 18 and 19, reflect this situation.

Of overriding importance is the necessity to administer adrenaline, at the dosages shown in the guidelines, immediately when the diagnosis is suspected. There is no time for delay. Even if the diagnosis is incorrect, in most instances intramuscular adrenaline is unlikely to cause any harm and so in general it is prudent to err on the side of caution. Once the adrenaline has been given, it is then important to lie the patient flat with the legs propped up (unless this is precluded by severe dyspnoea from bronchospasm). An intravenous line should be established where facilities exist.

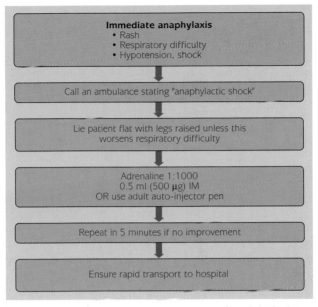

Figure 18. Anaphylactic reactions: treatment for adults in the community.

The effects of adrenaline will be abrogated in patients taking β-blockers. Nevertheless, some authorities recommend halving dosages of adrenaline stated in the guidelines for such patients because of a theoretical risk of unopposed α-adrenergic effects leading to hypertension and bradycardia. Similarly, halving the adrenaline dosages is also advocated by some inpatients taking amitryptyline and imipramine antidepressants, because these drugs inhibit noradrenaline reuptake. The desirability of these practices has yet to be ratified in appropriate trials. In the interim it is best to avoid such drugs in patients at risk of anaphylaxis.

Adrenaline reverses peripheral vasodilatation through its α-agonist effect, while its β-agonist effect dilates the airways, increases myocardial contractility and suppresses mast cell mediator release. In severe reactions, multiple

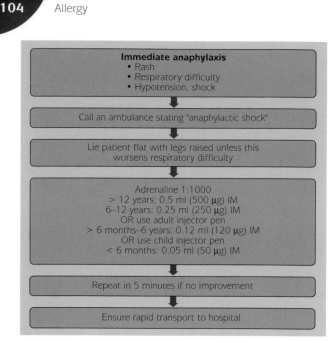

Figure 19. Anaphylactic reactions: treatment for children in the community.

dosages of adrenaline may be required. Injection intramuscularly into the thigh is recommended as the optimal site and route for adrenaline administration.[163,164] It should *not* be administered intravenously.

The only diagnostic test useful at the time of the reaction is measurement of the serum concentration of mast cell tryptase, which is usually, but not always elevated within 1–2 hours of a severe reaction. Elevated tryptase supports the diagnosis of an anaphylactic reaction if this is in doubt, but provides no information as to its mechanism or cause.

Follow-up management

A key aspect of the follow-up management of anaphylaxis is identification of the cause and subsequent avoidance. This should be managed by an experienced allergist. Careful enquiries as to all the possible causes of the anaphylactic episode should be pursued, as in Table 25. Foods, bee and wasp stings and drugs are common allergic causes. In many cases, the cause will be obvious or strongly suspected. Suspected allergic causes of anaphylaxis should be investigated further by appropriate skin prick testing or RAST. If the reaction has occurred during anaesthesia, appropriate guidelines should be followed by the anaesthetist (see *Drug allergy*). If a specific allergy is identified, it should be managed in its own right (see relevant sections). In some patients with recurrent anaphylaxis, a clear trigger factor is never uncovered.

The differential diagnosis of anaphylaxis includes other causes of urticaria, laryngeal oedema, bronchoconstriction and hypotension. Urticaria/angioedema directly caused by allergen exposure, as distinct from "idiopathic" disease, is usually obvious from the history (see *Urticaria/angioedema*). Acute laryngeal oedema and/or bronchospasm may be (and quite frequently are) mistaken for acute severe asthma. It is important to consider anaphylaxis as a cause of these symptoms, especially in patients not known to have asthma. Fainting, dizziness, hypotension and shock may also be caused by a wide variety of cardiological, neurological and metabolic diseases. Systemic mastocytosis, carcinoid syndrome and serum sickness should also be considered.

In cases where IgE-independent mechanisms are thought to be involved (see Table 25), appropriate challenge under supervision is sometimes indicated. In addition, because of the poor predictive value of positive skin prick tests, especially to foods, for allergic reactions, allergies suspected to have caused anaphylaxis from skin prick tests may also sometimes need verification by challenge. These procedures should be performed in specialist allergy centres with facilities for resuscitation and trained staff immediately available.

Patients at risk of repeated reactions from whatever cause should be provided with emergency medication tailored to fit their symptoms. This should be provided in a formal written plan that the patient understands. The plan may include antihistamines, short courses of oral steroids and inhaled bronchodilators. Regular non-sedating antihistamines, sometimes at supra therapeutic dosages, are often helpful for idiopathic disease where triggers cannot be avoided. Adrenaline aerosols such as Primatene Mist®, sprayed directly onto the mouth and tongue, can sometimes be useful in cases of severe lip and tongue swelling. All patients with life-threatening anaphylaxis should carry an adrenaline auto-injector pen.

Patients should be carefully instructed when and how to use such pens, and this training should be reiterated at intervals. Treatment plans should be sent to the appropriate occupational health supervisor at patients' workplaces. With children, the plan must be sent, with written parental permission, to the appropriate medical officer in the child's school. The local community paediatrician, who should be involved again with parental consent, commonly supervises treatment in schools. Medication and spare adrenaline pens should be available at work/school as well as at home.

Patient-based organizations, such as the Anaphylaxis Campaign in the UK, can be of enormous help to patients and their families (see Appendix 2).

Whenever possible, patients at risk of anaphylaxis should avoid taking β-blockers, ACE inhibitors, amitryptyline and imipramine (see earlier).

Urticaria and angioedema

Introduction

Urticaria ("hives", nettle rash) and angioedema (swelling of deeper, subcutaneous or submucosal tissue) are common disorders. They commonly occur together, but may occur separately. Urticaria usually reflects the release of histamine and other mast cell mediators, and consists of multiple, short-lived itchy swellings of the skin which are red and pale in the middle because of oedema, which then evolve into pink plaques which eventually disappear (Figure 20). They may vary in size from a few millimetres to several centimetres in diameter. Angioedema may also reflect histamine release, or the release of other mediators in immunological reactions resulting in increased capillary permeability and plasma leakage (Figure 21).

Figure 20. Typical urticarial rash.

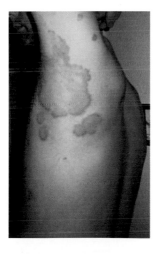

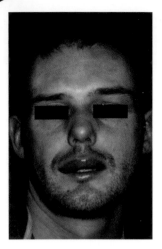

Figure 21. Typical angioedema of the upper lip and left upper eyelid.

Clinical classification

From the point of view of clinical diagnosis, the urticarial process may be classified as follows (Table 27).

Allergic reactions

In these cases the urticaria/angioedema is caused by classical, IgE-mediated mast cell degranulation. Symptoms occur reproducibly and typically within seconds or minutes after contact with an allergen to which the patient is sensitized. Reactions may be local or more generalized, depending on the patient's sensitivity. Common causes include:

- Following ingestion of foods in food allergic patients. Typical culprit foodstuffs (fresh fruits/vegetables, seafood, peanuts and tree nuts, milk and egg in infants) are often involved. The reactions occur immediately after ingestion of the food and not at any other time. They may be localized to the mouth and lips or more generalized. Severe reactions with generalized urticaria, bronchospasm, hypotension and laryngeal oedema may border on anaphylaxis.

Table 27. Clinical classification of urticaria/angioedema	
Classification	**Frequency in general practice***
Allergic urticaria/angioedema - food allergy - contact allergy - insect venom allergy - latex allergy - drug allergy	1–3%
Drug-induced urticaria/angioedema - aspirin/NSAIDs - ACE inhibitors - Other drugs	3–5%
Physical urticaria - cold urticaria - delayed pressure urticaria - cholinergic urticaria - solar urticaria - aquagenic urticaria - dermographism	5–10%
Idiopathic urticaria/angioedema - acute - chronic	85–95%
Hereditary angioedema	<< 1%
Underlying disease - vasculitis - cryoglobulinaemia - cold agglutinins - hypothyroidism	< 1%
*Approximate frequency of underlying cause in patients presenting to a general practitioner with urticaria/angioedema.	

- Following direct skin contact with an allergen (e.g. after picking up a cat or rolling in the grass) in patients allergic to these allergens.
- Following a bee or wasp sting in patients allergic to venom (again reactions may vary in severity and border on anaphylaxis).
- Following contact with latex in latex allergic individuals.

- Following ingestion of a drug, such a penicillin, to which the patient is allergic.

Such reactions account for only a small percentage of urticarial reactions seen in general practice. The diagnosis is generally obvious to the patient and the physician from a careful history. Occasionally, mild contact urticaria may be seen in the absence of IgE-mediated allergy, as in some patients who develop local urticaria after touching certain metals, preservatives and aerosolized substances such as adhesives or hairsprays.

Drug-induced urticaria

Although a wide variety of drugs may rarely cause urticaria/angioedema, the commonest culprits are aspirin and related NSAIDs and angiotensin converting enzyme (ACE) inhibitors. Aspirin-induced urticaria may be part of a general syndrome of aspirin sensitivity which may include aspirin-induced asthma, rhinitis and gastrointestinal upset. This is due to overproduction of leukotrienes. ACE inhibitors prevent the breakdown of kinins in the skin, causing angioedema in some patients. The effects of aspirin/NSAIDs and ACE inhibitors may be broadly cumulative, lowering the individual "urticarial threshold" in some patients.

Physical urticaria

In some patients mast cell degranulation in the skin may be caused by physical stimuli, which include the following conditions.

Cold urticaria. Patients experience a rapid onset of urticaria in contact with cold objects or after walking out in the cold, especially in exposed parts of the skin (face, neck and hands) on rewarming. The "ice-cube" test (where urticaria occurs under an ice-cube placed on the skin) is helpful in diagnosis. This is usually a benign disease, affecting young patients, more often females, although symptoms are occasionally systemic and severe. Rarely, secondary, cold urticaria in older patients may be caused by circulating cryoglobulins or cold agglutinins (see further).

Delayed pressure urticaria. Lesions appear where pressure has been applied to the skin (on the legs and buttocks after prolonged sitting in a chair, or on the soles of the feet after a long walk). The swelling is often delayed (3 7 hours after the pressure) and deeper and more painful than usual. Onset is typically in patients in their 30s and intermittent attacks may persist for years. Some patients feel unwell during attacks with fever, arthralgia and fatigue. This sort of urticaria often responds poorly to anti-histamines, and oral steroid therapy is sometimes necessary.

Cholinergic urticaria. Symptoms of urticaria appear when the body temperature rises because of overheating, exercise, stress or eating spicy foods.

Solar urticaria caused by exposure to bright sunlight.

Aquagenic urticaria caused by contact with water, swimming, baths and showers.

Dermographism. In this condition, the urticarial lesion may be induced locally by light stroking of the skin with a nail or another blunt instrument with application of pressure. The resulting wheal is itchy and linear, and arises within minutes and persists for several hours. This is a common disease in patients of all ages, and lasts 2 to 3 years. It often co-exists with other forms of idiopathic or physical urticaria. It may cause false-positive skin prick tests.

Vibratory angioedema caused by holding tools or other objects which vibrate.

The mechanisms of these generally benign reactions are poorly understood.[165]

Idiopathic urticaria/angioedema

Idiopathic disease constitutes up to 95% of the cases of urticaria/angioedema seen by a general practitioner. Symptoms are caused by apparently spontaneous mast cell degranulation. No external trigger factors are involved, and it is considered futile to search for these. There exists evidence that the disease is "autoimmune" in some patients who produce antibodies against the high-affinity IgE receptor on mast cells, which are then cross-linked by the antibodies, simulating IgE-mediated activation. Although frequently very frightening for patients when it first occurs, this disease is benign and self-limiting. Attacks may resolve within 6 weeks (acute idiopathic urticaria) but are frequently more prolonged (chronic idiopathic urticaria), although they usually wane both in frequency and severity with time. The median duration of the disease is 2–3 years, although 20% of patients continue to have minor, grumbling attacks for as long as 10 years.

Hereditary angioedema. This is caused by inherited, genetic deficiency of C1 esterase inhibitor, a protein which inhibits spontaneous activation of the complement cascade. Spontaneous activation of complement causes vascular leakage and angioedema (but, since there is no histamine release, never causes urticaria). The disease is very rare and inherited in an autosomal dominant fashion, so that a family history in first-degree relatives is the rule. Angioedema may involve the skin but more frequently involves intra-abdominal organs, causing acute abdominal pain and bowel obstruction. It may also occasionally cause laryngeal oedema, which can be fatal.

Manifestation of an underlying disease. Urticaria may rarely be a presenting feature of hypothyroidism or reflect the presence of circulating cold agglutinins or cryoglobulins, or underlying vasculitis caused by a variety of acute (e.g. following streptococcal sore throat) or chronic (e.g. systemic lupus erythematosus) diseases. Cold agglutinins and cryoglobulins may reflect underlying lymphoma or myeloma, or be produced in response to some chronic viral infections (such as hepatitis B or C). In addition, lympho-proliferative disease, particularly monoclonal gammopathy of undetermined significance (which may later progress to lymphoma or myeloma) may be associated with circulating auto-antibodies against C1 esterase inhibitor, causing proteolysis and consumption. Patients with cold agglutinins or cryoglobulins may have symptoms on exposure to cold, resembling benign cold urticaria (see earlier). Urticaria as a manifestation of such diseases is very rarely seen in general practice, but must not be missed. Danger signals, which should alert the physician to the possibility of these diseases, include:

- The urticaria/angioedema is relentless rather than evanescent and self-limiting, and painful rather than itchy.
- The skin shows evidence of residual petechial haemorrhage because of vasculitis (benign idiopathic and physical urticarias never leave any enduring marks on the skin).
- The patients have symptoms and signs of the underlying disease (patients with physical, allergic and idiopathic urticaria are otherwise fit and well, and remain so).
- Blood tests are abnormal (depending on the disease, one may observe elevated erythrocyte sedimentation rate (ESR), low thyroxine, deranged blood white cell counts, paraprotein bands on serum electrophoresis, positive auto-antibodies, positive cryoglobulins, positive hepatitis B or C serology): patients with physical or idiopathic urticaria have no abnormal blood tests.

Diagnosis

As with all allergy diagnosis, a careful and comprehensive clinical history is the key, since the diagnosis is essentially clinical.[166] Structured questionnaires to aid arrival at the correct diagnosis have been drawn up and are sometimes helpful.[167] It should be remembered that 95% or more of the cases presenting to the GP will comprise benign acute or chronic idiopathic disease, or physical urticaria. In idiopathic urticaria, the patient will typically have tried in vain to identify a precipitating cause. Specific enquiry should be made about the allergic causes of the disease in sensitized patients. Such patients will report acute and reproducible symptoms after exposure to the offending allergen (see earlier), and not at any other time, and the diagnosis should be obvious. More extensive enquiry should then be made as to the severity of allergic reactions, especially to foods, drugs, latex and bee or wasp stings (is there associated dizziness or fainting suggesting hypotension, bronchospasm or "closing of the throat" suggesting laryngeal oedema?).

A careful drug history should be taken, with special reference to aspirin, NSAIDs and ACE inhibitors. A simple diagnostic procedure is to stop the offending drug(s), and await resolution of the symptoms. Suitable replacement drugs may be necessary. For mild analgesia, paracetamol is a suitable alternative in most patients with aspirin-induced urticaria. Alternatively, the newer anti-inflammatory COX-2 inhibitor drugs such as rofecoxib are often tolerated. These drugs do not substitute for the anti-platelet effects of aspirin. In such cases, alternative anti-platelet drugs such as clopidogrel may be helpful. As substitutes for ACE inhibitors, drugs that block the angiotensin II receptor or alternative antihypertensive agents can be used.

Evidence should be sought about physical factors inducing the urticaria (see earlier). If hereditary angioedema is suspected, a family history is important. If an underlying disease is suspected (see "warning signs" earlier), then careful enquiry should be made about additional symptoms.

Laboratory testing

In cases of idiopathic and physical urticaria, which comprise more than 95% of cases presenting to a general practitioner, investigations of any sort are unnecessary. A systematic review of 29 studies including 6,462 patients presenting with idiopathic urticaria[4] revealed underlying disease in only 1.6% of patients (mostly connective tissue diseases or thyroid disease), so any blood test should be reserved for those few patients in whom an underlying disease is suspected from the history. These tests may include full blood count, ESR, thyroid function, differential white cell count and, in rare cases, auto-antibodies, serum electrophoresis, cryoglobulin and cold agglutinin tests or viral serology (see earlier).

In patients suspected of having urticaria as part of an acute reaction to allergen exposure, the diagnosis may be ratified by skin prick testing or RAST with the suspected allergen. Such patients should be referred to an allergist for further evaluation and management.

Patients with hereditary angioedema will have abnormal C1 esterase inhibitor activity (measured in hospital laboratories using a functional assay), and low serum concentrations of complement C4. While these patients should not be missed (and are difficult to miss given their very distinctive history and family history), it is pointless to perform these tests indiscriminately on all patients presenting with angioedema, particularly when it is associated with urticaria.

Management

The development of acute or chronic idiopathic urticaria/angioedema, occurring as it does "out of the blue" and causing widespread itchy rash and swelling of the face and limbs, can be a very frightening experience for patients; they will typically first present to an A&E department. Information and reassurance are therefore keystones of management. Physical and idiopathic urticaria are benign diseases[168] which remit spontaneously. The only "cure" is time. Patients must be informed of the likely chronic duration of the disease, and explained that it tends to remit, does not cause permanent damage to the skin or any other organ, and does not signal any form of underlying illness. Patients will often wrongly convince themselves that the disease is caused by a variety of environmental factors such as detergents, clothing or "something they have eaten": aside from true, immediate food allergic reactions, it must be explained to patients that such fears are unfounded and that they need not change their lifestyles in any way. Patients should be advised to avoid obvious physical trigger factors for urticaria as listed earlier. There is little to be gained from referring these patients to hospital, save for additional moral support for the patient or his/her primary care physician. Referral in these circumstances would normally be to a dermatologist.

Urticaria caused by an acute allergic reaction to foods, insect venom, drugs or latex should be managed in its own right by an allergist. It is particularly important to refer patients with symptoms and signs of severe allergic reactions suggesting borderline anaphylaxis (see earlier). Management includes avoidance of the offending allergen and other measures according to the nature of the allergen and the patient's sensitivity (see relevant sections).

Patients with suspected underlying diseases such as vasculitis should be referred to an appropriate specialist, (usually a rheumatologist, haematologist or immunologist) for further investigation and management. Patients with hereditary angioedema should be managed by a specialist allergist, immunologist or dermatologist.

Pharmacological management

Oral antihistamines are the main stay of drug therapy for chronic idiopathic and physical urticaria. Most patients respond well or at least partially to these drugs, which may be given regularly or intermittently according to the frequency and severity of symptoms. For routine daily use, non-sedating antihistamines are preferable (including cetirizine/levocetirizine, loratadine/desloratadine and fexofenadine). In adults, dosages in excess of the recommended therapeutic dosages are often used with good effect. For inexplicable reasons, some patients seem to do better with particular antihistamines, so it is worth trying different drugs if the initial response is unsatisfactory. Sedating antihistamines such as chlorpheniramine may be prescribed for troublesome symptoms at night, although these drugs may cause residual drowsiness the following day. Doxepin has antidepressant, as well as antihistamine and sedating properties and is useful for nocturnal therapy in some patients. Not all antihistamines are licensed to be used in infants and children, and dosages in children should be as licensed. Few types of antihistamine are recommended by their manufacturers for use in pregnancy: only chlorpheniramine and clemastine are considered safe, but are unfortunately sedating.

Adrenaline aerosols such as Primatene Mist®, sprayed directly onto the mouth and tongue, can sometimes be useful in cases of severe lip- and tongue-swelling. Oral steroids may useful for short periods especially for severe attacks, and in some forms of physical urticaria where antihistamines have a less marked effect. Short courses of prednisolone or equivalent (for example 30 mg for 5 days) may be used, and occasionally small regular dosages of prednisolone are justified. Oral steroids are perfectly safe in pregnancy.

If idiopathic or physical disease becomes severe, prolonged and intractable, further, more experimental types of therapy may be tried, usually under the supervision of a dermatologist. These include intravenous immunoglobulin therapy, PUVA therapy and immunosuppressive drugs such cyclosporin A and mycophenolate mofetil. With very few exceptions, these patients are at little risk of significant systemic reactions, and the prescription of adrenaline auto-injector pens is inappropriate. Hereditary angioedema may be managed prophylactically with danazol or, where this is unsuitable, acute attacks can be treated with infusions of fresh frozen plasma or purified C1 esterase inhibitor. Recombinant inhibitor is becoming available. These drugs should be administered under the management of an allergist or a dermatologist.

Allergen immunotherapy

Introduction

Specific allergen immunotherapy is defined as the administration of incremental dosages of relevant allergen in order to achieve clinical tolerance to the effects of allergen exposure. It was first described by Noon and Freeman, two English physicians, at the turn of the last century.[169] It is most used for seasonal atopic rhinoconjunctivitis (hayfever) and *Hymenoptera* venom-induced anaphylaxis. Its place in the treatment of perennial atopic rhinitis and atopic asthma remains controversial. It has not been found useful for the treatment of atopic dermatitis, urticaria and food allergy (in the last case, this reflects difficulty in defining and purifying food allergens in sufficient quantities). Although allergens are conventionally administered by subcutaneous injection, other methods of administration are being investigated.

Immunotherapy for allergic rhinoconjunctivitis

The efficacy and relative safety of immunotherapy for seasonal allergic rhinitis caused by tree or grass pollen allergy is not in doubt, and has been confirmed in a number of controlled clinical studies by various investigators including one of the authors of this volume[170,171] (Figure 22). It reduces both symptoms and medication usage, but it does not always abolish the need for some medical treatment during the pollen season. The place of immunotherapy in the management of patients with perennial allergic rhinitis caused by sensitivity to house dust mite or animal dander is less clear. Controlled trials of immunotherapy with house dust mite and animal dander have shown a statistical, if not clinically striking efficacy, but the procedure may benefit carefully selected patients.[172-174]

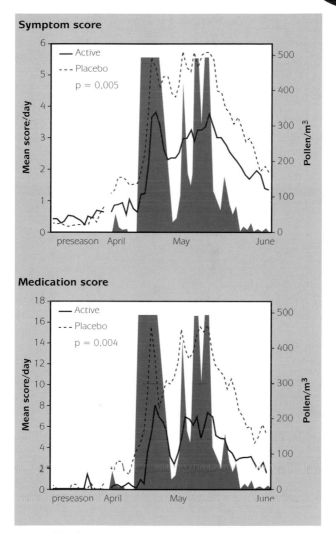

Figure 22. Symptom and medication scores in patients with rhinoconjunctivitis caused by birch pollen allergy treated for two years with birch allergen immunotherapy or placebo.
Reproduced with permission from Arvidsson MB *et al*. Effect of 2-year-placebo-controlled immunotherapy on airway symptoms and medication in patients with birch pollen allergy. *J Allergy Clin Immunol* 2002; **109**: 777–783.[170]

The duration of benefit is not precisely known but seems to be at least 6 years.[175]

Immunotherapy for atopic asthma

The role of immunotherapy in the management of atopic asthma is regarded in the UK as controversial. For this reason it has not so far been incorporated into the UK asthma therapy guidelines, despite its extensive use for asthma elsewhere. This discrepancy in the UK arises partly from a report issued by the Committee on Safety of Medicines in 1986 on fatalities and adverse reactions associated with immunotherapy,[176] most of which occurred in asthmatics. This led to the imposition of stringent restrictions on the practice of immunotherapy in the UK, effectively curtailing its administration in primary care. It has since become clear that allergen immunotherapy is safe if administered in a safe environment by experienced allergists trained to adjust dosages appropriately and to recognise and treat unwanted effects rapidly. Nevertheless, there is increased risk in asthmatics and, in general, only patients with documented mild and stable disease are eligible for treatment (see later).

Another problem with immunotherapy for atopic asthma is its efficacy in relation to conventional asthma therapy. Meta-analysis of placebo-controlled trials of immunotherapy with pollen and cat allergy-associated asthma[177] has shown a small but significant improvement in symptoms and lung function, but as might be expected these effects are very allergen-specific and best demonstrated when the particular allergen plays a clear role in exacerbation of asthma symptoms. Treatment with mixtures of allergens based on the results of skin prick tests alone is not effective.[178] Immunotherapy does not obviate the need for conventional asthma therapy, and it has not been shown to reduce therapy requirements.

Recent very important observations suggest that children with seasonal rhinoconjunctivitis treated with pollen immunotherapy are less likely to develop asthma[179] and new allergic sensitizations,[180] as compared with untreated children. If ratified, these data mean that immunotherapy is the only treatment which has so far been shown to alter favourably the natural history of progression of allergic disease, and this may result in its use being more widely recommended.

Immunotherapy for *hymenoptera* sensitivity

Immunotherapy is extremely effective for the therapy of severe systemic reactions caused by wasp and bee venom allergy. A full account is provided in *Insect venom allergy*.

Immunotherapy in clinical practice

Indications

Correct selection of patients for immunotherapy is of the utmost importance. Immunotherapy is offered to adults and older children with severe seasonal or perennial rhinoconjunctivitis who:

- Have a positive skin prick test and/or RAST to the relevant allergen
- Have a convincing history of allergen exposure causing symptoms
- Have severe disease despite a valid trial of medical therapy and allergen avoidance where possible.

Patients who do best are those with severe seasonal symptoms caused by grass or tree pollen allergy and those who are monosensitized to the causative allergen. Patients with both tree and grass pollen allergy can be desensitized concurrently (see further). In patients with perennial rhinoconjunctivitis sensitized to house dust mite, it is often difficult to ascertain that house dust mite exposure is responsible for the symptoms; nevertheless, immunotherapy is administered if symptoms are intractable despite avoidance and medical therapy. In patients with allergy to animal dander, immunotherapy is usually given if acute, severe symptoms are caused by unwanted exposure to animals (e.g. in the houses of friends), or if exposure is an occupational hazard (e.g. vets, animal welfare officers).

Patients should be able to make an informed decision to undergo immunotherapy with the advice of an experienced allergist. In general, mild symptoms can be treated adequately with pharmacotherapy. Many patients develop the impression that pharmacotherapy is ineffective because they do not understand that topical nasal steroids have no immediate effect in relieving symptoms, and that they must be taken regularly all year round for perennial symptoms, or starting a few weeks before the allergy the season to relive seasonal symptoms. Severe allergic conjunctivitis, which is often difficult to treat, may require immunotherapy. Some patients insist on immunotherapy because of its sustained, disease-modifying effect, and because they are reluctant to take drugs indefinitely. Unfortunately, immunotherapy does not always obviate the need for medical therapy.

The time commitment involved on behalf of the patient (and his/her physician) is also a consideration, since "standard" immunotherapy regimens last at least 3 years. Because of the paucity of allergy clinics currently in the UK, patients may have to travel considerable distances to receive treatment. (For bee and wasp venom immunotherapy, see *Insect venom allergy*).

Allergen extracts and regimens

Three principal forms of allergen extracts are used for immunotherapy (Table 28). Aqueous preparations are more easily standardized but more likely to cause systemic reactions. They are used for venom immunotherapy and "rush" schedules (this is explained later). In widely used depot preparations, the allergen is bound to a carrier – typically aluminium hydroxide or tyrosine – from which it is slowly released, producing fewer adverse reactions. Allergens chemically modified with methoxy-polyethylene glycol or formaldehyde or glutaraldehyde (allergoids), which are claimed to have reduced allergenicity, are increasingly used. It should be noted that only bee and wasp venom aqueous preparations (Pharmalgen®) and

Table 28. Advantages and disadvantages of available allergen preparations			
Allergen Preparation	**Advantages**	**Disadvantages**	**Principal uses**
Aqueous[*]	More easily standardized	Rapid absorption increases likelihood of unwanted effects	Widely used in USA; in Europe restricted to venom AI and for "rush" schedules
Depot (adsorbed to carrier such as aluminium hydroxide)	Slow release results in fewer unwanted effects	More difficult to standardize	Widely used in Europe, particularly for inhaled allergens
Chemically modified (a) mPEG modified extracts (b) Formaldehyde or glutaraldehyde modified extracts (allergoids)	At least in theory, show reduced allergenicity while retaining immunogenicity		Appear to be effective but not yet established in routine clinical use

[*]Following CSM restrictions, the only extracts currently routinely available for clinical use in the UK are aqueous bee and wasp venom extracts and tyrosine adsorbed tree and grass pollen.
mPEG = methoxy-polyethylene glycol, AI = allergen immunotherapy

tyrosine-adsorbed tree and grass pollen preparations (Pollinex®) are currently licensed for immunotherapy in the UK. All other preparations must be given on a "named patient" basis. Because allergens are currently standardized biologically, different manufacturers use their own units of biological activity of allergens. This makes it extremely difficult to transfer from one product to another. This problem should be eliminated when it is possible to manufacture allergens by recombinant DNA technology and standard dosages of allergens are defined universally.

Conventional immunotherapy regimens typically comprise an induction phase, where injections are given weekly for 8–12 weeks in incremental dosages, and a maintenance phase where the attained maintenance dosage is repeated, usually monthly (Table 29). Commonly, the

Table 29. Example of a "conventional" Allergen Immunotherapy schedule			
Week number	[Allergen] (µg/ml)	Dosage (ml)	Total allergen injected (µg)
Induction			
1	0.1	0.1	0.01
2	1	0.1	0.1
3	10	0.1	1
4	10	0.5	5
5	100	0.1	10
6	100	0.2	20
7	100	0.3	30
8	100	0.4	40
9	100	0.5	50
10	100	0.6	60
11	100	0.8	80
12	100	1	100
Maintenance			
13–150*	100	1	100

*There is no clear consensus as to the total duration of therapy. Empirically, 3 years of treatment have been recommended for allergies in general, although this may have to be prolonged if sensitivity (for example to venom) persists. Dosages are administered once or twice weekly during induction, and 4–6 weekly during maintenance.

total duration of treatment is 3 years, but this interval is arbitrary and subject to ongoing evaluation. The maintenance dosage of allergen is, again, not universally defined and depends on the nature of the allergen extract. Immunotherapy for pollens is usually started out of season. If the patient is receiving immunotherapy against more than one allergen, such as tree and grass pollen, induction for the second allergen may be started when the maintenance dosage of the first allergen is attained.

Conventional regimens are very time-consuming for patients and staff, and a number of shortened or "rush" regimens have been described in which the induction course is condensed into a short period, usually a few days. More details may be found in the European position paper on immunotherapy.[181]

Clinical considerations

Allergen injection should be given in a dedicated clinic, usually an allergy clinic, where facilities for the treatment of anaphylaxis, resuscitation equipment and trained staff are immediately available. At each visit, patients should be reviewed by an experienced allergist, who should document any intercurrent illness, changes in medication, recent exacerbations of disease and any unexpected exposure to allergen. The patient should be asked if there was any delayed reaction to the previous allergen injection. If any such risk factors are present, the allergist must consider either omitting the planned injection or modifying the dosage. PEF is monitored before, and 1 hour following, injections. The dosage of allergen administered should be cross-checked by two people. Allergens are administered slowly subcutaneously, and care must be taken to avoid intravenous injection. The recommended site for injections is the lateral aspect of the forearm.

According to European guidance,[181] immunotherapy with aeroallergens is absolutely contraindicated in:

- Patients with concurrent cardiac, immunopathological or malignant disease
- Patients taking monoamine oxidase inhibitors or β-blockers
- Patients considered unlikely to comply with the treatment regimen.

Immunotherapy is not currently recommended for:

- Children under the age of 5 years
- Pregnant women (although in some cases it may be appropriate to continue treatment if the patient becomes pregnant after treatment has started)
- Patients with severe dermatitis.

In the UK, immunotherapy is not recommended for the treatment of asthma, but may be given to patients with mild asthma, (PEF/forced expiratory volume [FEV_1] > 85% predicted), particularly seasonal asthma caused by pollen allergy, with *documented* evidence of stable disease (PEF charts). Contraindications to insect venom immunotherapy are discussed in *Insect venom allergy*.

Unwanted effects

Patients must be carefully observed following injection. Clinical evidence suggests that any severe systemic reactions will occur within 1 hour of injection.[182] For this reason, close observation in the clinic for 1 hour following all injections is mandatory. Severe systemic reactions must be treated with intramuscular adrenaline, antihistamines and intravenous fluids (see *Anaphylaxis*). Some degree of immediate local swelling occurs at the site of allergen injection in most patients, and rarely requires treatment. More severe local, and mild systemic reactions (rhinitis, erythema, urticaria and angioedema) may be treated with antihistamines prophylactically, if appropriate. These usually occur some hours following injection. Severe systemic reactions are very uncommon, occurring in 1% or fewer of all injections, commonly in the induction phase. A detailed consideration of adverse reactions to immunotherapy may be found in the BSACI position paper.[182]

Mechanism of action of immunotherapy

A variety of immunological changes has been described in association with immunotherapy,[183] but it remains uncertain which, if any, of these is responsible for the relief of symptoms.

Specific IgE

Allergen-specific IgE concentrations in the serum tend to increase early in the course of immunotherapy but subsequently decline. As observed in most studies, the clinical benefit is already apparent within the first 3 weeks, and therefore changes in allergen-specific IgE concentrations, at least in the serum, do not appear to be relevant to the mechanism of action of immunotherapy.

Specific IgG

Serum concentrations of allergen-specific IgG, particularly IgG$_4$, increase during immunotherapy as expected with any vaccination regimen. It has been suggested that this IgG acts as "blocking antibody", but there is little evidence to support this theory.

Cells and cytokines

Allergen immunotherapy may change the net cytokine profile of allergen-specific T cells. Successful immunotherapy is associated with increased T cell activation and local production of anti-allergic Th1-type cytokines, such as IFN-γ and IL-12, in target organs such as the skin and nose.[184] However, it is not clear how this phenomenon precisely relates to improvement of symptoms and reduced allergen reactivity of target organs.

Regulatory T cells

In addition to altering the cytokine profile of T cells, recent evidence suggests that immunotherapy may induce the production of allergen-specific regulatory T cells producing inhibitory cytokines such as IL-10 and TGF-γ.[185] These cells "turn off" the production of allergy-promoting cytokines by effector T cells in an allergen-specific fashion, reducing the numbers and activation of mast cells and eosinophils in the target organs.[175]

Novel modes of administration

Immunotherapy by direct application of allergen solutions to the nasal or buccal mucosa has been described as an alternative to allergen injection. Allergen concentrations much higher than those used for injection immunotherapy are used, and early trials suggest some efficacy with negligible unwanted effects.[186] However, compared with conventional immunotherapy, the efficacy and duration of action of the new procedures, as well as optimal duration of therapy, are yet to be determined.

With the advent of recombinant allergen technology, it has become possible to manufacture modified allergens which modulate T cell responses but are incapable of binding to allergen-specific IgE. These allergens therefore potentially increase the benefit/risk ratio of immunotherapy. A similar approach is to administer immunotherapy with allergen-derived peptides which affect T cell responses but do not bind to IgE.

Another approach currently under investigation is the co-administration of allergens with "immunostimulatory" substances, such as killed *Mycobacterium vaccae* or CpG oligonucleotides, which stimulate a strong allergen-specific, Th1-type T cell response and may enhance the efficacy of conventional immunotherapy.

All of these approaches must be carefully evaluated in terms of efficacy and, above all, safety before they can be considered suitable for routine use in patients.

Unconventional theories and unproven methods

There is a body of opinion that a wide variety of physical, behavioural, cognitive, affective and emotional symptoms represent allergic "diseases" caused by environmental "allergens". Typically, these diseases comprise a long-standing pattern of numerous symptoms referable to many organ systems. Physical examination is typically normal. Proponents of these diseases claim that "conventional" tests for allergy are unreliable, and sometimes advocate unproven diagnostic techniques. In general, however, the diagnosis rests on subjective reports that symptoms are related to environmental exposures. Suspect agents have been purported to include foods, food additives, drugs, environmental chemicals, hormones, micro-organisms and even electromagnetic radiation.

Chronic fatigue syndrome

Chronic fatigue syndrome, also called "allergic toxaemia" or "tension fatigue syndrome", is prototypical of this group of diseases. The symptoms are extremely variable but include recurrent headaches, abdominal pain, fatigue, muscle pain and respiratory complaints. The diagnosis has been made in both adults and children. Less frequent complications are said to include lymph node enlargement, fever, urinary frequency, colds, tachycardia, urticaria and difficulty in concentrating. The disease is often attributed to sensitivity to multiple foods, especially milk, chocolate and grains. The diagnosis is based solely on symptoms. Clinical examination and laboratory tests are typically normal, even for features that could be confirmed objectively. The onset of particular symptoms following food ingestion is typically delayed by hours, days or even weeks, and various dietary manipulations, usually performed extensively by patients, result in at best temporary relief, which usually leads to further dietary restriction.

To date, no definitive double-blind, placebo-controlled clinical trials have been offered in support of the existence of this syndrome. There is no evidence that therapeutic elimination diets successfully control symptoms.

Food additive sensitivity

This has been claimed to cause attention deficit hyperactivity disorder or "hyperactive" children. This is a behavioural condition characterized by excessive activity, lack of attention, difficulty with discipline and poor performance of children at school. The suggestion that this might be an allergic disorder was first raised by Feingold in 1973, based on the fact that one of his patients had aspirin-sensitivity and showed improvement of asthma and a range of unspecified psychiatric symptoms when placed on a salicylate-free diet. Based on these observations, Feingold recommended elimination of dietary salicylates for other psychiatric conditions.[187] Because of reports that asthmatic attacks in aspirin-sensitive asthmatics could be triggered by food colourings such as tartrazine,[188] he later recommended elimination of salicylates, as well as all food dyes and additives from the diet. In practice, complete salicylate avoidance in the diet is impossible. The few trials that have addressed the impact of dietary elimination or food colouring challenge have suffered from problems with patient selection, measurement of behavioural changes and blinding. Currently there is no evidence that toxicity, idiosyncratic reactions or metabolic hypersensitivity to food additives causes any direct effects on the central nervous system.[189]

Multiple food and chemical sensitivities: clinical ecology

The concept that certain individuals suffer a specific illness caused by multiple food and chemical sensitivities is the basis of the medical practice known as "clinical ecology". This disease has been known by several names previously, including environmentally induced disease, multiple chemical sensitivity, cerebral allergy and total allergy syndrome (for a review, see reference 190).

In 1996, a workshop organised by the World Health Organization[191] suggested a new name, "idiopathic environmental intolerance" (IEI), because the term "multiple chemical sensitivity" made an "unsupported assumption on causation", did not refer to a "clinically defined disease", and was not "based on validated clinical criteria for diagnosis".

IEI is described by clinical ecologists as a condition of multiple symptoms affecting numerous areas of the body without abnormal physical findings or conventional laboratory tests. Many complaints (commonly fatigue, headache, nausea, malaise, pain, mucosal irritation, dizziness) are non-specific.[192] The list of items claimed to cause these symptoms is essentially unlimited, and may include any foodstuff (including water itself), food additives of any type and almost any synthetic product or chemical, but particularly petrochemicals, solvents and paints. In many cases, patients complain of problems in public places such as public buildings or shopping precincts. Other cited causes have included natural gas, viruses, fungi, wood dust and occasionally endogenous hormones such as progesterone. These "causes" are said both to induce and to maintain the disease. There is no consistent relationship of symptoms to duration and degree of exposure. In addition, some well-defined medical illnesses such a rheumatoid arthritis, multiple sclerosis and irritable syndrome disease, as well as some psychiatric disorders, have been attributed to multiple food and chemical sensitivity.[192-194] Diagnostic procedures commonly include an extensive environmental history and the "provocation-neutralization" test (see later). Even without this test, a patient's self-report of symptoms occurring after presumed exposure to environmental odours, fumes or foods is usually sufficient to make the diagnosis. Following provocation-neutralization testing, patients commonly develop a new list of "causes" additional to the items used in the test.[192,195] The diagnosis may often be supported by validated laboratory tests including quantification of immunoglobulins or complement components, auto-antibodies, lymphocyte subsets and measurement of a variety of chemicals in blood, urine, fat and hair samples. Data from the clinical ecology literature and from independent review of a series of patients with IEI has lent no support to the diagnostic usefulness of any of these tests in IEI.[195]

Patients are often invited to take vitamin and mineral supplements, and some are given certain salts such as sodium bicarbonate, or even intravenous immunoglobulin or oxygen inhalation. Avoidance of multiple environmental chemicals is often recommended, which often necessitates a very significant change in lifestyle. Dietary manipulation usually includes avoidance of additives. A recent review of the response to this sort of therapy in a series of 50 cases[192] showed that in 2 years only two patients improved, 22 were unchanged and 26 were worse.

Patients will typically have consulted several specialists before finding their way to an allergist. They are frequently diagnosed by non-clinical ecologists as having somatization illness, anxiety, depression or hyperventilation. Some have been noted to display psychiatric features of post-traumatic stress disorder, agoraphobia, panic disorder and abuse in childhood. Formal studies[196] have suggested that the incidence of such diseases is higher than in controls, although a substantial proportion of patients show no significant psychiatric stress. Unfortunately, most patients are reluctant to accept a psychiatric diagnosis as a cause of their symptoms.

A pragmatic approach would involve abroad assessment of the patient with appropriate investigations, attention to any psychiatric disorder and help to restore physical and social functioning. The extent of medical investigation requires careful thought, since continued instigation of unproductive tests will reinforce the patient's belief that organic disease is present. Cognitive behavioural therapy shows some promise in IEI.[197] This is focused on illness beliefs and avoidance behaviour, with graded exposure to expected triggers.

Candida (yeast) hypersensitivity syndrome

This is based on a theory first forwarded by Truss that certain people develop hypersensitivity to a "toxin" released from *Candida albicans* that normally colonizes the gastrointestinal tract and vagina.[198] As with IEI, the possible symptoms are diverse and, typically, there are no physical findings or laboratory abnormalities (the disease should not be confused with infectious candidiasis or thrush, which occurs as a manifestation of many diseases, such as diabetes mellitus, or in the immunosuppressed). Many patients self-diagnose from books written for lay readers. Again, the *Candida* hypersensitivity syndrome has been claimed to be a precipitating or potentiating factor for many other diseases including arthritis, multiple sclerosis, schizophrenia, AIDS, depression and various emotional problems. Proponents often claim that the disease is caused by past exposure to antibiotics, steroids and sugars. There is no evidence to support such claims. The diagnosis is based entirely on the patients' history. Management consists of restriction of dietary sugars and yeast and foods claimed to contain moulds. Patients are often asked to take vitamin and mineral supplements, and may be treated with low dosages of oral anti-fungal agents such as nystatin, ketoconazole and occasionally amphotericin B.

The American Academy of Asthma, Allergy and Immunology has published a number of position statements regarding unconventional "allergic" diseases and unproven diagnostic techniques.[199-201]

Unproven diagnostic tests

A number of diagnostic tests that are not helpful for the diagnosis and management of allergy, but which continue to be advocated for this purpose, is shown in Table 30.

Table 30. Unproven diagnostic procedures in allergy

Advocated for	Procedure	Comments
Leukocytotoxic test Diagnosis of food allergy and sometimes inhalant allergy	Peripheral white blood cells suspended in sterile water and serum. Placed on a microscope slide previously coated with suspect food. Cells viewed microscopically for up to 2 hours. Various morphological changes used as evidence of "cytotoxicity".	Allergen-induced release of mediators is unlikely to be detected. No other clear scientific rationale. Results do not correlate with clinical illnesses.[197]
Provocation - neutralization "Allergy" to food and inhalant allergens and environmental chemicals (clinical ecology)	Intracutaneous injection with five-fold serial dilutions of allergen or chemical extracts. Patient records any and all subjective symptoms over the ensuing 10 minutes. If no symptoms are noticed, the dosage is increased until they are, then reduced until they are just not felt any more: the so-called "neutralizing" dosage.	Protocols are not standardized. No agreement about the significance of any local reactions. Every substance must be tested separately. In a blinded study patients could not distinguish active extracts from placebo.
Electrodermal testing (Vega testing) Claimed to identify food allergies	Uses a galvanometer to measure electrical resistance between two "acupuncture" points on the skin. The patient holds one electrode in the hand and the other is placed in various positions said to relate to specific allergies. Vials of food extracts contact an aluminium plate placed within the circuit.	This bizarre procedure has no theoretical basis and the results are empirical.[205,206]

Table 30. Unproven diagnostic procedures in allergy (cont.)		
Advocated for	Procedure	Comments
Applied kinesiology Claimed to identify "allergies"	Allergens in containers are held in one hand while a technician subjectively estimates the muscle strength in the opposite arm. A decrease in muscle power is said to indicate a positive test. For uncooperative infants a surrogate is tested, first alone then holding the child's hand.	There is no credible mechanistic basis for this test, and no scientific support that it is of any value.
Pulse test Allergy to various substances (most often foods)	A change in pulse rate (decrease or increase) after the ingestion, injection or sublingual application of a test substance. A change in pulse rate of 10 beats/min or more 15–20 minutes after exposure is said to be positive.	No valid theory or clinical evidence to support this test.
Hair analysis Claimed to assess health and nutritional status	Mineral analysis is performed in hair from near the scalp using unstandardized tests.	No evidence that low hair concentrations reflect low body stores. Influenced by age, gender, hairdyes and bleaches.
NuTron test Claimed to detect food intolerance and Candida sensitivity	Blood is incubated with in-house solutions of foodstuffs and neutrophil activation detected in a haematology analyser.	No validation or research evidence to support such claims

Many of these tests are available, often for a considerable fee, in high street stores, pharmacies and health food shops. These tests are at best unhelpful, and at worst potentially misleading and harmful (e.g. if they result in uninformed and inappropriate avoidance of foods to the extent of malnutrition). Even validated tests such as skin prick tests and the measurement of allergen-specific IgE (the latter test is also available by post from pharmacies and private diagnostic laboratories) are of limited worth unless interpreted in the light of the patients' history by an experienced allergist.

Some clinical laboratories also provide quantitative measurements of circulating IgG antibodies to food allergens. Again these are available to the public in stores and by post from websites. Although some have postulated that IgG antibodies may be responsible for delayed symptoms or other intolerance reactions to foods, there is as yet no evidence to support this hypothesis. It is known that low concentrations of food-specific IgG antibodies, detected by modern sensitive tests, circulate in normal individuals, but to date these are of no known pathogenetic significance.[202]

Unproven methods of treatment

A number of procedures in the realm of complementary medicine has been advocated for the treatment of allergic diseases, in addition to a wide variety of other diseases. A review of the evidence base, such as it exists, for several of these methods of treatment has recently been published by a group of its practitioners.[203]

Neutralization therapy is an extension of the provocation-neutralization testing procedure used in clinical ecology. After such testing, "neutralizing" doses of one or more substances are then self-administered by the patient using various routes. There are no established protocols. Practitioners of acupuncture recommend its use for the treatment of all forms of allergic disease. Such claims are scientifically unproven. Homoeopathy is based on the philosophy that "like cures like". This is translated into the administration of exceedingly minute quantities of substances believed to cause disease as a method of curing the disease. These substances are called "remedies" and usually consist of high dilutions of various natural extracts. The remedies are given orally. Homoeopaths claim to be able to cure numerous diseases, including all forms of allergic disease. There are few valid clinical studies to support this claim, although there is some evidence that the effects of homoeopathy are not attributable solely to placebo.[203]

Hazards of complementary and alternative medicine

Treatment is always a matter of balancing intended benefits to patients against risks of unwanted effects of therapy. This benefit/risk balance has been emphasised throughout this volume. It should be noted that complementary medicine is likewise not without risks. A recent review[204] documents cases of:

- Contact sensitivity to herbal preparations
- Anaphylactic reactions to grass pollen mixtures eaten as health foods
- Mechanical injuries (pneumothorax, cardiac tamponade) and infections (HIV, hepatitis) from acupuncture
- Contamination of herbal medicines with organophosphorus insecticides
- Deliberate adulteration of "natural" medicines with corticosteroids.

While these episodes are necessarily anecdotal (in the absence of any systematized reporting system for adverse effects of complementary medicines) and may be relatively rare, they do stress the need for caution, particularly when psychological dependence on a particular practice is also a problem.

Frequently asked questions

What is allergy?
Allergy is an abnormal, exaggerated response of the body's immune system to proteins (called allergens), which are inhaled into the nose and lungs, are eaten or come in contact with the skin. The symptoms of allergy may be chronic (wheezing and chest tightness in asthma, chronic eczema, nasal blockage in hayfever) or acute (sudden wheezing in asthma, itching and sneezing in hayfever, and anaphylactic (reactions to drugs, foods, latex and other substances).

What causes acute allergic reactions?
As part of the allergic response, individuals make a specific antibody to allergens called IgE, which sticks to cells that are called mast cells found in the skin, nose, lungs and bowels. On allergen exposure, the IgE causes sudden release of histamine and other substances from mast cells, resulting in acute allergic symptoms (chest and throat tightness, nettle rash and skin swelling, itching and sneezing, low blood pressure and dizziness).

Why do only some people become allergic?
This is not known for certain but susceptibility is partly inherited in the genes (a child has a 60% chance of being allergic if both parents are allergic, but only a 5% chance if neither parent is allergic). The external environment probably also plays an important role (discussed further below).

What can I do to stop my child developing allergies?
A number of strategies are currently undergoing evaluation. A few studies suggest that probiotics ("friendly" bacteria) taken by mouth by children or by their breast-feeding mothers may help. In "at-risk" children (that is, those in

whom one or both of the parents is/are allergic), breast-feeding seems to be protective, as does feeding with a hydrolyzed infant milk formula. Delayed introduction of solid foods is also thought to be helpful in preventing food allergies (cow's milk and eggs should be avoided for at least 12 months, and nuts for 2 or 3 years if possible).

Is allergy on the increase?

The number of people with allergies continues to grow, and new allergies such as that to latex are on the increase. In any one year, over 20% of the population (12 million people) have an active allergic disease needing treatment. Currently, 6% of all general practice consultations are for allergic diseases. About one in 70 children now have allergic reactions to peanuts. Severe hayfever is one of the commonest causes of loss of time from school or work.

Why is allergy on the increase?

The recent rapid increase in allergies, particularly in developing countries, suggests that, in addition to genetic predisposition, environmental influences play an important role. One theory is that the reduction in childhood infections and in general exposure to dirt has let allergy develop. Changes in diet (too much junk food and not enough anti-oxidants) may also be relevant. Modern living conditions (stuffy, under-ventilated bedrooms with central heating and double-glazing) tend to increase indoor allergens. Certain aspects of pollution may be contributory, although overall pollution in general has fallen greatly in the last 50 years, whereas the incidence of allergy has risen. It is not certain which, if any, of these environmental factors are the most important.

I have hayfever but my nose runs and feels blocked all the year round. Why is this?

Such patients are probably allergic not only to grass or tree pollen but some other allergens (animal dander or house dust mite) that are present all year round. These patients should have allergy skin prick testing to provide a list of allergens that are clinically important. Avoidance advice can then follow.

Hayfever makes my life a misery. What can I do?

Firstly, such patients should see a GP or an allergist for skin prick testing to determine exactly what allergens are causing the symptoms. Secondly, these patients should be prepared to take a steroid nasal spray and an antihistamine tablet every day during the pollen season, commencing at least 2 or 3 weeks before the time at which symptoms usually start. Antihistamine eye drops for severe ocular symptoms may also help. Certain patients may be suitable for immunotherapy ("desensitization" injections: this should be discussed with an allergist).

My child has terrible eczema. Will allergen avoidance help?

It certainly may do. As far as possible, children should avoid contact with all indoor allergens to which they are clinically allergic, such as animal dander, house dust mite, pollens and moulds. In addition, up to 40% of young children with severe eczema have a food allergy, and avoidance of relevant foods can produce significant clinical improvement. This must be managed by an allergist and also sometimes by a dietician.

Do special diets help adults with severe eczema or asthma?

Unlike infants and young children, in whom avoidance of food allergens may improve asthma, eczema and rhinitis, in adults there is little evidence that dietary manipulation can alter the natural progression of eczema or asthma, or reduce the need for concurrent treatment. But of course, all patients with severe allergic reactions to certain foods, in particular asthmatics who are more at risk of severe bronchospasm, should avoid these foods.

How do I know if I have a food allergy?

True food allergies caused by allergic IgE antibodies generally cause reproducible and immediate reactions to the offending foodstuff. Typical culprits are dairy produce – especially in children – seafood, grains, nuts and, increasingly, fruit and vegetables. These reactions include: swelling and itching of the lips and tongue (oral allergy syndrome); itchy skin rash with swelling (urticaria or hives around the mouth, or generalized); sickness, vomiting and, in severe cases, hoarseness and closing up of the throat (laryngeal oedema); chest tightness and low blood pressure, which may cause dizziness and fainting (or clumsiness, drowsiness and inattention in infants).

Will my symptoms of food allergy get worse?

This is possible but unlikely. People vary in their allergic sensitivity to foods for reasons that we do not understand. Although reactions to foods such as peanuts may be severe, many more reactions are mild and remain so.

Can I be "screened" for food allergies?

No. This is not possible because skin prick tests and blood tests for food allergies are often positive even when there is no clinical allergic reaction. Allergy tests can only be used to confirm patients' suspicions of food allergies (that is, when they have reproducible symptoms of allergy, as listed earlier, on exposure to specific foods). In the absence of such a history, reactions to foods cannot be reliably predicted, although a negative skin prick test confirms that the possibility of any allergic reaction is extremely unlikely.

Is irritable bowel syndrome caused by food allergy?

No. Patients with irritable bowel syndrome do not usually have symptoms of food allergy. Some studies suggest that exclusion diets may be useful in irritable bowel syndrome, but the foods to avoid must be defined by trial and error and cannot be predicted by any allergy test. The disease is best managed by a gastroenterologist.

I am told that I developed a rash with given penicillin for a sore throat as a child. Does this mean that I am allergic to penicillin and cannot take it again?

There are two main kinds of allergic reaction to drugs. In the first and commonest case, a rash develops some hours or days after starting the drug. This is rarely, if ever, life-threatening and usually clears up when the drug is stopped. In the second and less common case, the body produces allergic IgE antibody against the drug, which means that a severe allergic reaction may develop if the drug is taken again. These two types of reaction are unconnected. In general, patients who have had delayed rashes after taking a drug like penicillin are no more likely than anyone else to produce IgE antibodies, and so the risk of a rapid, severe allergic reaction is low. In case of doubt, the results of a skin prick test with a solution of the drug can help to make decisions: a negative test provides reassurance that a severe allergic reaction is extremely unlikely; a positive test indicates that the patient may be at risk of severe allergic reactions and therefore suitable alternative drugs may be chosen.

Are there reliable tests for drug allergy?

Not as many as one would wish for. In patients who have had an immediate, severe allergic reaction to a drug, a positive skin prick test will confirm the suspected diagnosis of IgE-mediated drug allergy. However, many patients with a positive skin prick test to a drug will not develop any sort of reaction to it, so the test cannot be used in a prospective sense to predict response. More delayed reactions to drugs, such as rashes and disorders or renal or liver function, are not caused by IgE. At present, there are no tests available which can predict such reactions.

What is anaphylaxis?

Anaphylaxis is a severe allergic reaction caused by widespread release of histamine from mast cells around the body. Causes include food, drug, vaccine, bee and wasp sting, latex allergy and, occasionally, exercise. In some cases, the precipitating causes are hard to identify. Anaphylaxis is a potential danger to life because it may cause swelling of the larynx, which blocks the airways, causing severe worsening of asthma and extreme falls in blood pressure. Patients at risk should be carefully assessed by an allergist to determine and remove the cause of anaphylaxis, and should carry emergency medication (antihistamines, adrenaline injector pen and a written emergency action plan).

Who may be eligible for allergen immunotherapy?

There are two main categories of patients: those with bee or wasp venom allergy, and those with severe allergic rhinitis (usually summer hayfever caused by allergy to tree and/or grass pollens). It is important to recognize and refer patients with immediate systemic allergic reactions to bee or wasp stings, since immunotherapy in these patients is highly effective. It should be noted that patients with large local reactions to stings, whatever the size, do not qualify for treatment in the absence of a systemic reaction. The same applies to children in whom the natural history of the disease is benign and remission is usually rapid. Adults and children with severe hayfever who have failed to respond to properly administered medical therapy may benefit from immunotherapy and should be referred to an allergist.

Do patients with chronic urticaria/angioedema need allergy tests?

95% or more of cases of recurrent urticaria/angioedema seen in general practice are "idiopathic", that is, the attacks occur in the absence of any external allergen provocation. Most of these patients need no diagnostic investigations. The only cure for the disease is time, although regular or intermittent antihistamines help reduce the severity of the attacks. A small proportion of patients with urticaria/angioedema develop this as a part of an acute allergic reaction to an external allergen (following a bee or wasp sting, immediately after ingesting a particular food, on contact with latex, after touching a cat or other object to which the patient is sensitized). Drugs may also be responsible (aspirin and related non-steroidals, and angiotensin-converting enzyme (ACE) inhibitors are particular culprits). These patients do need further investigation by an allergist, especially if the resulting reaction is severe.

References

1. Royal College of Physicians. *Allergy: the unmet need. A blueprint for better patient care. Report of the Royal College of Physicians working party on the provision of allergy services in the UK.* London: Royal College of Physicians, June 2003.

2. Newson R, Strachan D, Archibald E, *et al.* Effect of thunderstorms and airborne grass pollen on the incidence of acute asthma in England, 1990–94. *Thorax* 1997; **52**: 680–685.

3. Emberlin J. The effects of air pollution on allergenic pollen. *Eur Respir Rev* 1998; **8**: 164–167.

4. Custovic A, Murray CS, Gore RB, Woodcock A. Environmental allergen control. *Ann Allergy Asthma Immunol* 2002; **88**: 432–441.

5. Robinson DS, Hamid Q, Ying S, *et al.* Predominant TH2-like bronchoalveolar T-lymphocyte population in atopic asthma. *N Engl J Med* 1992; **326**: 298–304.

6. Ray A, Cohn L. TH2 cells and GATA-3 in asthma: new insights into the regulation of airway inflammation, *J Clin Invest* 1999; **104**: 985–993.

7. Weller PF. The immunobiology of eosinophils. *N Engl J Med* 1991; **324**: 1110–1118.

8. Oettgen HC, Geha RS. IgE regulation and roles in asthma pathogenesis. *J Allergy Clin Immunol* 2001; **107**: 429–440.

9. Zlotnik A, Yoshie O. Chemokines: a new classification system and their role in immunity *Immunity* 2000; **12**: 121–127.

10. Wahn U, Von Mutius E. Childhood risk factors for atopy and the importance of early intervention. *J Allergy Clin Immunol* 2001; **107**: 567–74.

11. Illi S, Von Mutius E, Lau S, Nickel S *et al.* The pattern of atopic sensitisation is associated with the development of asthma in childhood. *J Allergy Clin Immunol* 2001; **108**: 709–714.

12. Sengler C, Lau S, Wahn U, Nickel R. Interactions between genes and environmental factors in asthma and atopy: new developments. *Respir Res* 2002; **3**: 7–34.

13. Martinez FD. What have we learned from the Tucson Children's Respiratory Study? *Paediatr Respir Rev* 2002; **3**: 193–197.

14. Custovic A, Simpson BM, Murray CS *et al*. The National Asthma Campaign Manchester Asthma and Allergy Study. *Pediatr Allergy Immunol* 2002; **13** (Suppl. 15): 32–37.

15. Umetsu DT, McIntire JJ, Akbari O *et al*. Asthma: an epidemic of dysregulated immunity. *Nature Immunol* 2002; **3**: 715–720.

16. Strachan DP. Hayfever, hygiene and household size. *BMJ* 1989; **299**:1259–1260.

17. Ball TM, Castro-Rodriguez JA, Griffith KA *et al*. Siblings, day-care attendance and the risk of asthma and wheezing during childhood. *N Engl J Med* 2000; **343**: 536–543.

18. Illi S, Von Mutius E, Lau S *et al*. Early childhood infectious diseases and the development of asthma up to school age: a birth cohort study. *BMJ* 2001; **322**: 390–395.

19. Matricardi PM, Rosmini F, Panetta V *et al*. Hayfever and asthma in relation to markers of infection in the United States. *J Allergy Clin Immunol* 2002; **110**: 381–387.

20. Braun-Fahrlander C, Gassner M, Grize L *et al*. Prevalence of hayfever and allergic sensitisation in farmer's children and their peers living in the same rural community: SCARPOL team Swiss Study on Childhood Allergy and Respiratory Symptoms with Respect to Air Pollution. *Clin Exp Allergy* 1999; **29**: 28–34.

21. von Mutius E, Braun-Fahrlander C, Schierl R *et al*. Exposure to endotoxin or other bacterial components might protect against the development of atopy. *Clin Exp Allergy* 2000; **30**: 1230–1234.

22. Zuany-Amorin C, Manlius C, Trifilieff A *et al*. Long-term protective and antigen-specific effect of heat-killed *Mycobacterium vaccae* in a murine model of allergic pulmonary inflammation. *J Immunol* 2002; **169**: 1492–1499.

23. Horner AA, Raz E. Immunostimulatory sequence oligodeoxynucleotide-based vaccination and immunomodulation: two unique but complementary strategies for treatment of allergic diseases. *J Allergy Clin Immunol* 2002; **100**: 706–712.

24. Loibichler C, Pichler J, Gerstmayr M *et al.* Materno-fetal passage of nutritive and inhaled allergens across placenta of term and pre-term deliveries perfused *in vitro*. *Clin Exp Allergy* 2002; **32**: 1546–1551.

25. Custovic A, Woodcock A. Exposure and sensitisation in infants and children. *Curr Opin Allergy Clin Immunol* 2001; **1**: 133–138.

26. Daniels SE, Bhattacharrya S, James A *et al.* A genome-wide search for quantitative trait loci underlying asthma. *Nature* 1996; **383**: 247–250.

27. Van Eerdewegh P, Little RD, Dupuis J *et al.* Association of the ADAM33 gene with asthma and bronchial hyperresponsiveness. *Nature* 2002; **418**: 426–430.

28. American Academy of Pediatrics. Committee on Nutrition. Hypoallergenic infant formulas. *Pediatrics* 2000; **106**: 346–349.

29. Holst A, Koletzko B, Dreborg S *et al.* Summary recommendations of the ESPACI Committee on hypoallergenic formulas and ESPGHAN Committee on Nutrition. *Arch Dis Child* 1999; **81**: 80–84.

30. Kalliomaki M, Salminen S, Arvilommi H *et al.* Probiotics in primary prevention of atopic disease: a randomised placebo-controlled trial. *Lancet* 2001; **357**: 1076–1079.

31. Faith-Magnusson K, Kjellman NI. Development of atopic disease in babies whose mothers were receiving exclusion diet during pregnancy: a randomised study. *J Allergy Clin Immunol* 1987; **80**: 868–875.

32. Gdalevich M, Mimouni D, David M. *et al.* Breastfeeding and the onset of atopic dermatitis in childhood: a systematic review and meta-analysis of prospective studies. *J Am Acad Dermatol* 2001; **45**: 520–527.

33. Gdalevich M, Mimouni D, Mimouni M. Breastfeeding and the risk of bronchial asthma in childhood: a systematic review with meta-analysis of prospective studies. *J Pediatr* 2001; **139**: 261–266.

34. Kramer MS, Kakuma. Maternal dietary antigen avoidance during pregnancy and/or lactation for preventing or treating atopic disease in the child (Cochrane Review). Cochrane Database of Systematic Reviews, CD000133. The Cochrane Library, Issue 4, 2003. Chichester: John Wiley & Sons Ltd.

35. Ram FSF, Ducharme FM, Scarlett J. Cow's milk protein avoidance and development of childhood wheeze in children with a family history of atopy (Cochrane Review). Cochrane Database of Systematic Reviews, CD003795. The Cochrane Library, Issue 4, 2003. Chichester: John Wiley & Sons Ltd.

36. American Academy of Pediatrics. Committee on Nutrition. Soy protein-based formulas: recommendations for use in infant feeding. *Pediatrics* 1998; **101**: 148–153.

37. Businco L, Dreborg S, Einarsson R *et al*. Hydrolysed cow's milk formulae. Allergenicity and use in treatment and prevention. An ESPACI position paper. European Society of Paediatric Allergy and Clinical Immunology. *Paediatr Allergy Immunol* 1993; **4**: 101–11.

38. von Berg A, Koletzko S, Grubl A *et al*. The effect of hydrolysed cow's milk formula for allergy prevention in the first year of life: the German Infant Nutritional Intervention Study, a randomised double-blind trial. *J Allergy Clin Immunol* 2003; **111**: 533–540.

39. Wilson AC, Forsyth JS, Greene SA *et al*. Relation of infant diet to childhood health: seven year follow up of cohort of children in Dundee infant feeding study. *BMJ* 1998; **316**: 21–25.

40. Anonymous. British guidelines on the management of asthma. *Thorax* 2003; **58**: (Suppl. 1): il–i94.

41. Kips JC, Pauwels RA. Long-acting inhaled beta(2)-agonist therapy in asthma. *Am J Respir Crit Care Med* 2001; **164**: 923–932.

42. Becker AB, Simons FE. Formoterol, a new long-acting selective beta 2-adrenergic receptor agonist: double-blind comparison with salbutamol and placebo in children with asthma. *J Allergy Clin Immunol* 1989; **84**: 891–895.

43. Ducharme FM, Hicks GC. Anti-leukotriene agents compared to inhaled corticosteroids in the mangement of recurrent and/or chronic asthma in adults and children (Cochrane Review). Cochrane Database of Systematic Reviews, CD002314. The Cochrane Library, Issue 4, 2003. Chichester: John Wiley & Sons Ltd.

44. Knorr B, Franchi LM, Bisgaard H, *et al.* Montelukast, a leukotriene receptor antagonist, for the treatment of persistent asthma in children aged 2 to 5 years. *Pediatrics* 2001; **108**: E48.

45. Adams NP, Bestall JB, Jones PW. Inhaled beclomethasone versus placebo for chronic asthma (Cochrane Review). Cochrane Database of Systematic Reviews, CD002314. The Cochrane Library, Issue 4, 2003. Chichester: John Wiley & Sons Ltd.

46. Adams N, Bestall J, Jones PW. Inhaled fluticasone proprionate for chronic asthma (Cochrane Review). Cochrane Database of Systematic Reviews, CD003135. The Cochrane Library, Issue 4, 2003. Chichester. John Wiley & Sons Ltd.

47. Brocklebank D, Ram F, Wright J *et al*. Comparison of the effectiveness of inhaler devices in asthma and chronic obstructive airways disease: a systematic review of the literature. *Health Technol Assess* 2001; **5**: 1–149.

48. Pearson MG, Bucknall CE, eds. *Measuring clinical outcome in asthma: a patient-focused approach*. London: Royal College of Physicians, 1999.

49. Gallefoss, F, Balle PS. Impact of patient education and self-management on morbidity in asthmatics and patients with chronic obstructive pulmonary disease. *Respir Med* 2000; **94**: 279–287.

50. Lahdensuo A, Haahtela T, Herrala J *et al.* Randomised comparison of guided self management and traditional treatment of asthma over one year. *BMJ* 1996; **312**: 748–752.

51. Wesseldine LJ, McCarthy P, Silverman M. Structured discharge procedure for children admitted to hospital with acute asthma: a randomised controlled trial of nursing practice. *Arch Dis Child* 1999; **80**: 110–114.

52. George MR, O'Dowd LC, Martin I *et al.* A comprehensive educational program improves clinical outcome measures in inner-city patients with asthma. *Arch Intern Med* 1999; **159**: 1710–1716.

53. Sporik R, Holgate ST, Platts-Mills TA *et al.* Exposure to house-dust mite allergen (Der p l) and the development of asthma in childhood. *N Engl J Med* 1990; **323**: 502–527.

54. Peat JK, Salome CM, Woolcock AJ. Longitudinal changes in atopy during a 4-year period: relation to bronchial hyperresponsiveness and respiratory symptoms in a population sample of Australian schoolchildren. *J Allergy Clin Immunol* 1990; **85**: 65–74.

55. Sherrill D, Stein R, Kurzius-Spencer M *et al.* Early sensitisation to allergens and development of respiratory symptoms. *Clin Exp Allergy* 1999; **29**: 905–911.

56. Platts-Mills TA, Thomas WR, Aalberse RC *et al.* Dust mite allergens and asthma: report of a second international workshop. *J Allergy Clin Immunol* 1992; **89**: 1046–1060.

57. Gotzsche PC, Hammarquist C, Burr M. House dust mite control measures in the management of asthma: meta-analysis. *BMJ* 1998; **317**: 1105–1110.

58. Gøtzsche PC, Johansen HK, Burr ML, Hammarquist C. House dust mite control measures for asthma (Cochrane Review). Cochrane Database of Systematic Reviews, CD001187. The Cochrane Library, Issue 4, 2003. Chichester: John Wiley & Sons Ltd.

59. Abramson M, Puy R, Weiner J. Immunotherapy in asthma: an updated systematic review. *Allergy* 1999; **54**: 1022–1041.

60. Ross RN, Nelson HS, Finegold I. Effectiveness of specific immunotherapy in the treatment of asthma: a meta-analysis of prospective, randomised, double-blind, placebo-controlled trials. *Clin Ther* 2000; **22**: 329–341.

61. Abramson MJ, Puy RM, Weiner JM. Allergen immunotherapy for asthma (Cochrane Review). Cochrane Database of Systematic Reviews, CD001186. The Cochrane Library, Issue 4, 2003. Chichester: John Wiley & Sons Ltd.

62. Pajno G, Barbero G, De Luca F *et al.* Prevention of new sensitisations in asthmatic children monosensitised to house dust mite by specific immunotherapy. *Clin Exp. Allergy* 2001; **31**: 1392–1397.

63. Dezateau C, Stocks J, Dundas I *et al.* Impaired airway function and wheezing in infancy: the influence of maternal smoking and a genetic predisposition to asthma. *Am J Respir Crit Care Med* 1999; **159**: 403–410.

64. Strachan DP, Cook DG. Health effects of passive smoking. 1. Parental smoking and lower respiratory illness in infancy and early childhood. *Thorax* 1997; **52**: 905–914.

65. Murray AB, Morrison BJ. The decrease in severity of asthma in children of parents who smoke since the parents have been exposing them to less cigarette smoke. *J Allergy Clin Immunol* 1999, **91**: 102–110.

66. Rasmussen F, Siersted HC, Lambrechtsen J *et al.* Impact of airway lability, atopy, and tobacco smoking on the development of asthma-like symptoms in asymptomatic teenagers. *Chest* 2000; **117**: 1330–1335.

67. Gannon PF, Weir DC, Robertson AS *et al.* Health, employment, and financial outcomes in workers with occupational asthma. *Br J Ind Med* 1993; **50**: 491–496.

68. Worldwide variation in prevalence of symptoms of asthma, rhinoconjunctivitis, and atopic eczema: ISAAC. The International Study of Asthma and Allergies in Childhood (ISAAC) Steering Committee. *Lancet* 1998; **351**: 1225–1232.

69. Wuthrich, B, Schindler C, Leunenberger P, Ackerman-Liebrich U. Prevalence of atopy and pollinosis in the adult population of Switzerland (SALPADIA study). Swiss Study on Air Pollution and Lung Diseases in Adults. *Int Arch Allergy Immunol* 1995; **106**: 149–156.

70. Bousquet J, Van Cauwenberge P, Khaltaev N. Aria Workshop Group, World Health Organization. Allergic Rhinitis and its impact on asthma. *J Allergy Clin Immunol* 2001; **108** (5 Suppl.): S147–S336.

71. van Cauwenberge P, Bachert C, Pasalacqua G *et al.* Consensus statement on the treatment of allergic rhinitis. Position paper. *Allergy* 2000; **55**: 116–134.

72. Togias A. Rhinitis and asthma: evidence for respiratory system integration. *J Allergy Clin Immunol* 2003; **111**: 1171–1183.

73. Settipane R, Hagy G, Settipane G. Long-term risk factors for developing asthma and allergic rhinitis: a 23-year follow-up study of college students. *Allergy Proc* 1994; **15**: 21–25.

74. Crystal-Peters J, Neslusan C, Crown WH, Torres A. Treating allergic rhinitis in patients with comorbid asthma: the risk of asthma-related hospitalisations and emergency department visits. *J Allergy Clin Immunol* 2002; **109**: 57–62.

75. Cuffel B, Warmboldt M, Borish L *et al.* Economic consequences of comorbid depression, anxiety and allergic rhinitis. *Psychosomatics* 1999; **40**: 491–496.

76. Schultz-Larsen F, Hanifin JM. Epidemiology of atopic dermatitis. *Immunol Allergy Clin North Am* 2002; **22**: 1–24.

77. Williams H, Robertson C, Stewart A *et al.* Worldwide variations in the prevalence of symptoms of atopic eczema in the International Study of Asthma and Allergies in Childhood. *J Allergy Clin Immunol* 1999; **103**: 125–138.

78. Sampson HA. Food allergy. Part 1. Immunopathogenesis and clinical disorders. *J Allergy Clin Immunol* 1999; **103**: 717–728.

79. Wheatley LM, Platts-Mills TAE. Role of inhalant allergens in atopic dermatitis. In: Leung DYM, Greaves MW, editors. *Allergic skin disease: a multi-disciplinary approach*, New York: Marcel Dekker, 2000.

80. Tan BB, Weald D, Strickland I *et al.* Double-blind controlled trial of effect of house dust-mite allergen avoidance on atopic dermatitis. *Lancet* 1996; **347**: 15–18.

81. Gutgesell C, Heise S, Seubert S *et al*. Double-blind placebo-controlled study off house dust mite control measures in adult patients with atopic dermatitis. *Br J Dermatol* 2001; **145**: 70–74.

82. Holm L, Bengtsson A, van Hage-Hamsten M *et al*. Effectiveness of occlusive bedding in the treatment of atopic dermatitis – a placebo-controlled trial of 12 months' duration. *Allergy* 2001; **56**: 152–158.

83. Leyden JJ, Kligman AM. The case for steroid-antibiotic combinations. *Br J Dermatol* 1977; **96**: 179–187.

84. Tzaneva S, Seeber A, Schwaiger M *et al*. High-dose versus medium-dose UVA1 phototherapy for patients with severe generalized atopic dermatitis. *J Am Acad Dermatol* 2001; **45**: 503–507.

85. Van Der Meer JB, Glazenburg EJ, Mulder PG *et al*. The management of moderate to severe atopic dermatitis in adults with topical fluticasone propionate. The Netherlands Adult Atopic Dermatitis Study Group. *Br J Dermatol* 1999; **140**: 1114–1121.

86. Reitamo S. Tacrolimus: a new topical immunomodulatory therapy for atopic dermatitis. *J Allergy Clin Immunol* 2001; **107**: 445–448.

87. Bock SA, Sampson HA, Atkins FM *et al*. Double blind, placebo-controlled food challenge (DPCFC) as an office procedure: a manual. *J Allergy Clin Immunol* 1988; **82**: 986–997.

88. Young E, Stoneham MD, Petruckevitch A *et al*. A population study of food intolerance. *Lancet* 1994; **343**: 1127–1130.

89. Hide DW, Guyer BM. Cow's milk intolerance in Isle of Wight infants. *Br J Clin Pract* 1983; **37**: 285–287.

90. Nickel R, Kulig M, Forster J *et al*. Sensitization to hen's egg at the age of twelve months is predictive for allergic sensitisation to common indoor and outdoor allergens at the age of 3 years. *J Allergy Clin Immunol* 1997; **99**: 613–617.

91. Sicherer SH, Munoz-Furlong A, Burks AW *et al*. Prevalence of peanut and tree nut allergy in the United States

of America. *J Allergy Clin Immunol* 1999; **103**: 559–562.

92. Young E, Stoneham MD, Petruckevitch A *et al*. A population study of food intolerance. *Lancet* 1994; **343**: 1127–1130.

93. Kanny G, Moneret-Vautrin DA, Flabbee J *et al*. Population study of food allergy in France. *J Allergy Clin Immunol* 2001; **108**: 133–140.

94. Tariq SM, Stevens M, Matthews W *et al*. Cohort study of peanut and tree nut sensitisation by age of 4 years. *BMJ* 1996; **313**: 514–517.

95. Grundy J, Matthews S, Bateman B *et al*. Rising prevalence of allergy to peanut in children: data from 2 sequential cohorts. *J Allergy Clin Immunol* 2002; **110**: 784–789.

96. ALSPAC website: http://www.alspac.bris.ac.uk/AlspacExt/

97. Chiu L, Sampson HA, Sicherer SH. Estimation of the sensitisation rate to peanut by prick skin test in the general population: results from the National Health and Nutrition Examination Survey 1988–94 (NHANES III). *J Allergy Clin Immunol* 2001; **107**: S192 (abstract).

98. Sampson HA, Scanlon SM. Natural history of food hypersensitivity in children with atopic dermatitis. *J Pediatr* 1989; **115**: 23–27.

99. Vander Leek TK, Liu AH, Stefanski K *et al*. The natural history of peanut allergy in young children and its association with serum peanut-specific IgE. *J Pediatr* 2000; **137**: 749–755.

100. Ewan PW. Clinical study of peanut and nut allergy in 62 consecutive patients: new features and associations. *BMJ* 1996; **312**: 1074–1078.

101. Pumphrey RS. Lessons for management of anaphylaxis from a study of fatal reactions. *Clin Exp Allergy* 2000; **30**: 1144–1150.

102. Alves B, Sheikh A. Age specific aetiology of anaphylaxis. *Arch Dis Child* 2001; **85**: 348.

103. Burks AW, Mallor SB, Williams L *et al*. Atopic dermatitis: clinical relevance of food hypersensitivity reactions. *J Pediatr*

1988; **113**: 447–451.

104. Onorato J, Merland N, Terral C *et al*. Placebo-controlled double-blind food challenge in asthma. *J Allergy Clin Immunol* 1986; **78**:1139–1146.

105. Hourihane JO, Dean TP, Warner JO. Peanut allergy in relation to heredity, maternal diet, and other atopic diseases: results of a questionnaire survey, skin prick testing and food challenges. *BMJ* 1996; **313**: 518–521.

106. Ewan PW, Clark AT. Long-term prospective observational study of the outcome of a management plan in patients with peanut and nut allergy referred to a regional allergy centre. *Lancet* 2001; **357**: 111.

107. Roberts G, Lack G. Food allergy: getting more out of your skin prick tests. *Clin Exp Allergy* 2000; **30**: 1495–1498.

108. Nanda R, James R, Smith H *et al*. Food intolerance and the irritable bowel syndrome. *Gut* 1989; **30**: 1099–1104.

109 Egger J, Carter CM, Soothill JF, Wilson J. Oligoantigenic diet treatment of children with epilepsy and migraine. *J Pediatr* 1989; **114**: 51–58.

110 Cars O, Molstad S, Melander A. Variation in antibiotic use in the European Union. *Lancet* 2001; **357**: 1851–1853.

111. Blanca M. Allergic reactions to penicillins. A changing world? *Allergy* 1995; **50**: 777–782.

112. The Association of Anaesthetists of Great Britain and Ireland and the British Society for Allergy and Clinical Immunology. *Suspected anaphylactic reactions associated with anaesthesia, 3rd edition*. London: The Association of Anaesthetists of Great Britain and Ireland and the British Society for Allergy and Clinical Immunology, 2003.

113. Nagel JE, White C, Lin MS *et al*. IgE synthesis in man. II. Comparison of tetanus and diphtheria IgE antibody in allergic and non-allergic children, *J Allergy Clin Immunol* 1979; **63**: 308–314.

114. Liberman P, Patterson R, Metz R *et al*. Allergic reactions to insulin. *JAMA* 1971; **215**: 1106–1112.

115. Retailliau HF Curtis AC, Storr G *et al*. Illness after influenza vaccination reported through a nationwide surveillance system, 1976–1977. *Am J Epidemiol* 1980; **111**: 270–278.

116. Nasser SM, Ewan PW. Opiate-sensitivity: clinical characteristics and the role of skin prick testing. *Clin Exp Allergy* 2001; **31**: 1014–1020.

117. Pichler WJ, Schnyder B, Zanni M *et al*. Role of T cells in drug allergies. *Allergy* 1998; **53**: 225–232.

118. Crockard AD, Ennis M. Laboratory-based allergy diagnosis: should we go with the flow? *Clin Exp Allergy* 2001; **31**: 975–977.

119. Beezhold D, Beck WC. Surgical glove powders bind latex allergens. *Archives of Surgery* 1992; **127**; 1354–1357.

120. Posch A, Wheeler C, Dunn MJ *et al*. Characterisation and identification of latex allergens by two-dimensional electrophoresis and protein microsequencing. *J Allergy Clin Immunol* 1997; **99**: 385–395.

121. Nutter AF. Contact Urticaria to rubber. *Br J Dermatol* 1979; **101**: 597–598.

122. Ownby DR, Ownby HE, McCullough J, Shafer AW. The prevalence of anti-latex IgE antibodies in 1000 volunteer blood donors. *J Allergy Clin Immunol* 1996; **97**: 1188–1192.

123. Merrett TG, Merrett J, Kekwick R. The prevalence of immunoglobulin E antibodies to the proteins of rubber (*Hevea brasiliensis*) latex and grass (*Phleum pratense*) pollen in sera of British blood donors. *Clin Exp Allergy* 1999; **29**: 1572–1578.

124. Saxon A, Ownby D, Huard T *et al.* Prevalence of IgE natural rubber latex in unselected blood donors and performance characteristics of AlaSTAT testing. *Ann Allergy Asthma Immunol* 2000; **84**: 199–206.

125. Gautrin D, Infante-Rivard C, Dao TV *et al*. Specific IgE-dependent sensitisation, atopy, and bronchial hyperresponsiveness in apprentices starting exposure in protein-derived agents. *Am J Resp Crit Care Med* 1997; **155**: 1841–1847.

126. Bernadini R, Novembre E, Ingargiola A *et al.* Prevalence and risk factors of latex sensitisation in an unselected pedriatic population. *J Allergy Clin Immunol* 1998; **101**: 621–625.

127. Liss GM, Sussman GL. Latex sensitisation: occupational versus general population prevalence rates. *Am J Ind Med* 1999; **35**: 196–200.

128. Pridgeon C, Wild G, Asthworth F *et al.* Assessment of latex allergy in a healthcare population: are the available tests valid? *Clin Exp Allergy* 2000; **30**: 1444–1449.

129. Heilman DK, Jones RT, Swanson MC *et al.* A prospective, controlled study showing that rubber gloves are the major contributor to latex aeroallergen levels in the operating room. *J Allergy Clin Immunol* 1996; **98**: 325–330.

130. Mazón A, Nieto A, Estornell F *et al.* Factors that influence the presence of symptoms caused by latex allergy in children with spina bifida. *J Allergy Clin Immunol* 1997; **99**: 600–604.

131. Blanco C, Carrillo T, Ortega N, *et al.* Comparison of skin-prick test and specific serum IgE determination for the diagnosis of latex allergy. *Clin Exp Allergy* 1998; **28**: 971–976.

132. Anonymous. Task force on allergic reactions to latex. American Academy of Allergy and Immunology. Committee Report. *J Allergy Clin Immunol* 1993; **92**: 16–18.

133. Slater JE. Latex allergy – what do we know? *J Allergy Clin Immunol* 1992; **3**: 279–281.

134. Gold M, Swartz JS, Braude BM *et al.* Intraoperative anaphylaxis: an association with latex sensitivity. *J Allergy Clin Immunol* 1991; **87**: 662–666.

135. The Association of Anaesthetists of Great Britian and Ireland and The British Society For Allergy and Clinical Immunology. *Suspected anaphylactic reactions associated with anaesthesia, 3rd revised edition.* London: The Association of Anaesthetists of Great Britian and Ireland and The British Society For Allergy and Clinical Immunology, 2003.

136. Laxenaire MC. Epidemiology of anaesthetic anaphylactoid reactions. Fourth multicenter survey (July 1994-December 1996). *Ann Fr Anesth Reanim* 1999; **18**: 796–809.

137. Holzman RS. Clinical management of latex-allergic children. *Anesth Analg* 1997; **85**: 529–533.

138. Dakin MJ, Yentis SM. Latex allergy: a strategy for management. *Anaesthesia* 1998; **53**: 774–781.

139. American Society of Anesthesiologists. Natural rubber latex allergy: considerations for anesthesiologists. American Society of Anesthesiologists 1999 (website: http://www.asahq.org).

140. Field EA, Longman LP, Al-Sharkawi M *et al.* The dental management of patients with natural rubber latex allergy. *Br Den J* 1998; **185**: 65–69.

141. Björnsson E, Janson C, Plaschke P *et al.* Venom allergy in adult Swedes: a population study. *Allergy* 1995; **50**: 800–805.

142. Hunt KJ, Valentin MD, Sobotka AK *et al.* A controlled trial of immunotherapy in insect hypersensitivity. *N Engl J Med* 1978; **299**: 157–161.

143. Valentin MD, Schuberth KC, Kagey-Sobotka A *et al.* The value of immunotherapy with venom in children with allergy to insect stings. *N Engl J Med* 1990; **323**: 1601–1603.

144. Golden DBK, Marsh DG, Friedhoff LR *et al.* Natural history of Hymenoptera venom sensitivity in adults. *J Allergy Clin Immunol* 1997; **100**: 760–766.

145. Ewan PW. Venom allergy. *BMJ* 1998; **316**: 1365–1368.

146. Egner W, Ward C, Brown DL, Ewan PW. The incidence and clinical significance of specific IgE to both wasp (Vespula) and bee (Apis) venom in the same patient. *Clin Exp Allergy* 1998; **26**: 26–34.

147. Golden DBK, Kagey-Sobotka A, Norman PS, Hamilton RG. Insect sting allergy with negative venom skin test responses. *J Allergy Clin Immunol* 2001; **107**: 897–901.

148. Muller UR. New developments in the diagnosis and treatment of hymenoptera venom allergy. *Int Arch Allergy Immunol* 2001; 124: 447–453.

149. Muller U, Mosbech H. Position papers: immunotherapy with Hymenoptera venoms. *Allergy* 1993; **48** (Suppl. 114): 37–46.

150. Oude Elberink JNG, de Monchy JGR, Golden DBK *et al*. Development and validation of a health-related qualify-of-life questionnaire in patients with yellow jacket allergy. *J Allergy Clin Immunol* 2002; **109**: 162–170.

151. Anonymous. Position paper on allergen immunotherapy. Report of a BSACI working party. January–October 1992. *Clin Exp Allergy* 1993; **23** (Suppl. 3): 1–44.

152. McHugh SM, Deighton J, Steward AG *et al*. Bee venom immunotherapy induces a shift in cytokine responses from a TH2 to a TH1 dominant pattern: comparison of rush and conventional therapy. *Clin Exp Allergy* 1995; **25**: 828–38.

153. Nasser SM, Ying S, Meng Q, *et al*. Interleukin-10 levels increase in cutaneous biopsies of patients undergoing wasp venom immunotherapy. *Eur J Immunol* 2001; **31**: 3704–3713.

154. Ewan PW. New insight into immunological mechanisms of venom immunotherapy. *Curr Opinion Allergy Immunol* 2001; **1**: 367–374.

155. Kemp SF. Anaphylaxis: a review of causes and mechanisms. *J Allergy Clin Immunol* 2002; **110**: 341–348.

156. Sampson HA. Anaphylaxis and Emergency Treatment. *Pediatrics* 2003; **111**: 1601–1608.

157. Stewart AG, Ewan PW. The incidence, aetiology and management of anaphylaxis presenting to an Accident & Emergency department. *QJM* 1996; **89**: 859– 864.

158. Yunginger JW. Anaphylaxis. *Annals of Allergy* 1992; **69**: 87–97.

159. Sheikh A, Alves B. Hospital admissions for acute anaphylaxis: time trend study. *BMJ* 2000; **320**: 1441.

160. Project Team of the Resuscitation Council (UK). Emergency medical treatment of anaphylactic reactions. *J Accid Emerg Med* 1999; **16**: 243–248.

161. Project Team of the Resuscitation Council (UK). The emergency medical treatment of anaphylactic reactions. *Resuscitation* 1999; **41**: 93–99.

162. Project Team of the Resuscitation Council (UK). Update on the emergency medical treatment of anaphylactic reactions for the first medical responders and for community nurses. *Resuscitation* 2001; **48**: 241–243.

163. Simmons FER, Gu X, Simons KJ. Epinephrine absorption in adults: Intramuscular versus subcutaneous injection. *J Allergy Clin Immunol* 2001; **108**: 871–873.

164. Simmons FER, Roerts JR, Gu X, Simons KJ. Epinephrine absorption in children with history of anaphylaxis. *J Allergy Clin Immunol* 1998; **101**: 33–337.

165. Gratan CEH, Sabroe RA, Greaves MW. Chronic urticaria. *J Am Acad Dermatol* 2002; **46**: 645–457.

166. Kozel MMA, Mekkes JR, Bossuyt PMM, Bos JD. The effectiveness of history based diagnostic approach in chronic urticaria and angioedema. *Arch Dermatol* 1998; **134**: 1575–1580.

167. Kozel MMA, Ansari Moein MC, Mekkes J *et al*. Evaluation of clinical guidance for the diagnoses of physical and chronic urticaria and angioedema. *Acta Derm Venereol* 2002; **82**: 270–274.

168. Kozel MMA, Bossuyt PMM, Mekkes JR, Bos JD. Laboratory tests and identified diagnoses in patients with physical and chronic urticaria and angioedema: a systematic review. *J Acad Dermatol* 2003; **48**: 409–416.

169. Noon L. Prophylactic inoculation against hay-fever. *Lancet* 1919; **1**:1572–1573.

170. Arvidsson MB, Löwhagen O, Rak S. Effect of 2-year placebo-controlled immunotherapy on airway symptoms and medication in patients with birch pollen allergy. *J Allergy Clin Immunol* 2002; **109**: 777–783.

171. Varney VA, Gaga M, Frew AJ *et al*. Usefulness of immunotherapy in patients with severe summer hay fever uncontrolled by anti-allergic drugs. *BMJ* 1991; **302**: 265–269.

172. Carrado OJ, Pastorello E, Ollier S *et al*. A double-blind study of hyposensitisation with an alginate conjugated extract of *D. pteronyssinus* ("Conjuvac") in patients with perennial rhinitis. *Allergy* 1989; **44**: 108–115.

173. Bousquet J. Lockey F, Malling HJ. Allergen immunotherapy: therapeutic vaccines for allergic diseases. A WHO position paper. *Allergy* 1998; **102** (4 Pt 1): 558–562.

174. Varney VA, Edwards J, Tabbah K *et al.* Clinical efficacy of specific immunotherapy to cat dander: a double-blind placebo-controlled trial. *Clin Exp Allergy* 1997; **27**: 860–867.

175. Varga EM, Durham SR. Allergen injection immunotherapy. *Clin Allergy Immunol* 2002; **16**: 533–549.

176. Committee on the Safety of Medicines. CSM update: desensitising vaccines. *Brit Med J* 1986; **293**: 948.

177. Abramson MJ, Puy RM, Weiner JM. Allergen immunotherapy for asthma (Cochrane Review). In: The Cochrane Library, Issue 4, 2003. Chichester: John Wiley & Sons Ltd.

178. Adkinson NF, Egleston PA, Eney D *et al.* A controlled trial of immunotherapy for asthma in allergic children. *N Engl J Med* 1997; **336**: 324–331.

179. Möller C, Dreborg S, Ferdousi IIA *et al.* Pollen immunotherapy reduces the development of asthma in children with seasonal rhinoconjunctivitis (the PAT-study). *J Allergy Clin Immunol* 2002; **109**: 251–256.

180. Des Roches A, Paradis L, Menardo JL *et al.* Immunotherapy with a standardized Dermatophagoides pteronyssinus extract. VI. Specific immunotherapy prevents the onset of new sensitisations in children. *J Allergy Clin Immunol* 1997; **99**: 450–453.

181. Malling HJ, Weeke B. Revised EAACI position paper on immunotherapy. *Allergy* 1993; **48** (Suppl 14): 9–35.

182. Position paper on allergen immunotherapy. Report of a BSACI Working Party. *Clin Exp Allergy* 1993; **23** (Suppl. 3): 1–44.

183. Frew AJ. Immunotherapy of allergic disease. *J Allergy Clin Immunol* 2003; **111** (2 Suppl.): S712–719.

184. Hamid QA, Schotman E, Jacobson MR *et al.* Increases in IL-12 messenger RNA+ cells accompany inhibition of allergen-induced late skin responses after successful grass pollen immunotherapy. *J Allergy Clin Immunol* 1997; **99**: 254–260.

185. Francis JN, Till SJ, Durham SR. Induction of IL-10+CD4+CD25+ T cells by grass pollen immunotherapy. *J Allergy Clin Immunol* 2003; **111**: 1255–1261.

186. Nelson HS. Advances in upper airway diseases and allergen immunotherapy. *J Allergy Clin Immunol* 2003; **111** (3 Suppl.): S793–S798.

187. Feingold BF. *Why your child is hyperactive*. New York: Random House, 1975.

188. Chafee FH, Settipane GA. Asthma caused by FD&C approved dyes. *J Allergy* 1967; **40**: 65–72.

189. Consensus Conference: defined diets and childhood hyperactivity. *JAMA* 1982; **248**: 290–292.

190. Reid S. Multiple chemical sensitivity – is the environment really to blame? *J Royal Soc Med* 1999; **92**: 616–619.

191. United Nations Environment Program – International Labor Office – World Health Organization. Conclusions and recommendations of a workshop on multiple chemical sensitivities (MCS). *Regul Toxicol Pharmacol* 1996; **24**: 188–189.

192. Terr AI. Environmental illness. A clinical review of 50 cases. *Arch Intern Med* 1986; **146**: 145–149.

193. Monro J, Carini C, Brostoff J. Migraine is an allergic disease. *Lancet* 1984; **2**: 719–721.

194. Simon GE, Katon WK, Sparks PJ. Allergic to life: psychological factors in environmental illness. *Am J Psychiatry* 1990; **147**: 901–906.

195. Terr AI. Clinical ecology in the workplace. *J Occup Med* 1989; **31**: 257–261.

196. Black DW, Rathe A, Goldstein RB. Environmental illness. A controlled study of 26 subjects with "20th century disease." *JAMA* 1990; **264**: 3166–3170.

197. Stenn P, Binkley K. Successful outcome in a patient with chemical sensitivity. *Psychosomatics* 1998; **39**: 547–50.

198. Truss CO. Tissue injury induced by *Candida albicans:* mental and neurologic manifestations. *J Orthomol Psy* 1978; **7**: 1–19.

199. Anonymous. American Academy of Allergy and Immunology: position statements – controversial techniques. *J Allergy Clin Immunol* 1981; **67**: 333–334.

200. Anonymous. Clinical ecology. Executive Committee of the American Academy of Allergy and Immunology. *J Allergy Clin Immunol* 1986; **78**: 269–271.

201. Anonymous. Candidiasis hypersensitivity syndrome. Executive Committee of the American Academy of Allergy and Immunology. *J Allergy Clin Immunol* 1986; **78**: 271–273.

202. Sheffer AL, Lieberman PL, Aaronson DW *et al.* Measurement of circulating IgG and IgE food-immune complexes. *J Allergy Clin Immunol* 1988; **81**: 758–760.

203. Lewith GT, Breen A, Filshie J, Fisher P *et al.* Complementary medicine: evidence base, competence to practice and regulation. *Clin Med* 2003; **3**: 235–240.

204. Niggemann B, Gruber C. Side effects of complementary and alternative medicine. *Allergy* 2003; **58**: 707–716.

205. Lewith GT, Kenyon JN, Broomfield J *et al.* Is electrodermal testing as effective as skin prick tests for diagnosing allergies? A double-blind, randomised block design study. *BMJ* 2001; **332**: 131–134.

206. Semizzi M, Senna G, Crivellaro M, Rapacioli G *et al.* A double-blind, placebo-controlled study on the diagnostic accuracy of an electrodermal test in allergic subjects. *Clin Exp Allergy* 2002; **32**: 928–32.

Appendix 1 – Drugs

Drug	Format	Trade name	Preparation	Strengths	Dosages	Comments	Side effects
Inhaled short-acting β-agonists for asthma							
Salbutamol	Oral	Generic	Tablet	2 mg, 4 mg	Up to 16 mg daily (children 2–12 yr 8 mg) divided in 4 dosages	Not generally recommended for asthma (see *Asthma*)	Tremor Tachycardia Hypokalaemia Headache Insomnia
			Solution	2 mg/5 ml			
		Ventolin	Syrup	2 mg/5 ml			
		Ventmax SR	Capsule	4 mg	8 mg (children 3–12 yr 4 mg) twice daily		
		Volmax	Tablet	4 mg			
	Inhalation	Generic	MDI	100 µg/puff	100–200 µg up to 4 times daily	Used as a short-term reliever for asthma: overusage suggests poor asthma control (see *Asthma*)	
			DPI	200 µg/puff			
		Cyclocaps for Cyclohaler	DPI	200 µg, 400 µg/puff			
		Airomir	MDI	100 µg/puff			
		Airomir Autohaler	BAMDI	100 µg/puff			
		Asmasal Clickhaler	BAMDI	95 µg/puff			
		Salamol Easi-Breathe	BAMDI	100 µg/puff			
		Ventodisks for Diskhaler	DPI	200 µg/puff			

Drug	Format	Trade name	Preparation	Strengths	Dosages	Comments	Side effects
Inhaled short-acting β-agonists for asthma							
Salbutamol	Inhalation	Ventolin Accuhaler	DPI	200 µg/puff	100–200 µg up to 4 times daily	Used as a short-term reliever for asthma: overusage suggests poor asthma control (see *Asthma*)	Tremor Tachycardia Hypokalaemia Headache Insomnia
		Ventolin Evohaler	MDI	100 µg/puff			
	Nebulized	Generic	Nebulizer solution	2.5 mg, 5 mg	2.5 mg (children < 18 mo 1.25 mg) up to 4 times daily		
		Ventolin	Nebule				
Terbutaline sulphate	Oral	Bricanyl	Tablet	5 mg	Up to 15 mg (children < 7 yr up to 2.25 mg, > 7 yr up to 7.5 mg) daily divided in 3 dosages	Not generally recommended for asthma (see *Asthma*)	Tremor Tachycardia Hypokalaemia Headache Insomnia
		Bricanyl	Syrup	1.5 mg/5 ml			
		Monovent	Syrup	1.5 mg/5 ml			
		Bricanyl SA	Tablet	7.5 mg	7.5 mg twice daily		
	Inhalation	Bricanyl	MDI	250 µg/puff	250–500 µg up to 4 times daily	Used as short-term reliever for asthma	
		Bricanyl Turbohaler	DPI	500 µg/puff			
	Nebulized	Generic	Nebulizer solution	5 mg	Up to 10 mg up to 4 times daily (reduce in children)		
		Bricanyl	Respule	5 mg			

Drug	Format	Trade name	Preparation	Strengths	Dosages	Comments	Side effects
Inhaled long-acting β-agonists for asthma							
Formeterol fumarate	Inhalation	Foradil	DPI	12 µg/puff	12 µg or 24 µg twice daily adults and children > 6 yr	First-line "add-on" asthma therapy at step 3 of therapy (see *Asthma*)	As for SABA. Occasionally cause paradoxical bronchospasm. Care with formoterol in liver disease and pregnancy.
		Oxis Turbohaler	DPI	6 µg, 12 µg/ puff			
Salmeterol xinafoate	Inhalation	Serevent Accuhaler	DPI	50 µg/puff	Adults and children >4 yr 50 µg or 100 µg twice daily.		
		Serevent Diskhaler	DPI	50 µg/puff			
		Serevent MDI	MDI	25 µg/puff			
Antimuscarinic bronchodilators for asthma							
Ipratropium bromide	Inhalation	Atrovent	DPI	40 µg/puff	20–40 µg up to 4 times daily (children < 6 yr up to 20 µg, > 6 yr up to 40 µg 3 times daily)	4th or 5th-line therapy in asthma at Steps 4 and 5 of treatment (see *Asthma*). Duration of action 3–6 hr.	Use with caution in glaucoma, prostatism, pregnancy, breast-feeding. Dry mouth, nausea, constipation, headache.
		Aerocaps for Aerohaler	DPI				
		Atrovent MDI	MDI	20 µg/puff	DPI not recommended in children < 12 yr		
		Atrovent Forte MDI	MDI	40 µg/puff			
		Atrovent Autohaler	BAMDI	20 µg/puff			

Drug	Format	Trade name	Preparation	Strengths	Dosages	Comments	Side effects
Antimuscarinic bronchodilators for asthma							
Oxitropium bromide	Inhalation	Oxivent MDI	MDI	100 µg/puff	200 µg/puff 2–3 times daily	4th or 5th-line therapy in asthma at Steps 4 and 5 of treatment (see *Asthma*).	Use with caution in glaucoma, prostatism, pregnancy, breast feeding.
		Oxivent Autohaler	BAMDI	100 µg/puff	Not recommended in children	Duration of action 3–6 hr.	Dry mouth, nausea, constipation, headache.
Methylxanthines for asthma							
Theophylline	Oral	Nuelin	Tablet	125 mg	125 mg 3–4 times daily (reduce in children)	Brand must be specified. 2nd or 3rd-line "add-on" therapy in patients with asthma at Step 3 or above (see *Asthma*).	Tachycardia, palpitations, nausea, headache, insomnia.
			Liquid	60 mg/5 ml			Plasma concentrations must be monitored (therapeutic range 10–20 mg/l).
		Nuelin SA	Tablet	175mg	175–350 mg every 12 hr	Aminophylline infusion is also used for acute severe asthma but **not** without plasma levels in patients taking oral theophylline or aminophylline.	Clearance affected by liver disease, cardiac failure, old age and many other drugs.
		Nuelin SA 250	Tablet	250mg	250–500 mg every 12 hr		
		Slo-phyllin	Capsule	60 mg, 125 mg, 250 mg	250–500 mg every 12 hr (reduce in children)		
		Uniphyllin Continus	Tablet	200 mg, 300 mg, 400 mg	200–400 mg every 12 hr (children 9 mg/kg every 12 hr)		

Methylxanthines for asthma

Drug	Format	Trade name	Preparation	Strengths	Dosages	Comments	Side effects
Aminophylline	Oral	Generic	Tablet	100 mg	100–200 mg 3–4 times daily	Brand must be specified. 2nd or 3rd-line "add-on" thereapy in patients with asthma at Step 3 or above (see *Asthma*). Aminophylline infusion is also used for acute severe asthma but **not** without plasma levels in patients taking oral theophylline or aminophylline.	Tachycardia, palpitations, nausea, headache, insomnia. Plasma concentrations must be monitored (therapeutic range 10–20 mg/l). Clearance affected by liver disease, cardiac failure, old age and many other drugs.
		Phyllocontin Continus	Tablet	225 mg	225–450 mg twice daily		
		Forte	Tablet	350 mg			
		Paediatric	Tablet	100 mg	Up to 12 mg/kg twice daily		

Inhaled corticosteroids for asthma

Drug	Format	Trade name	Preparation	Strengths	Dosages	Comments	Side effects
Beclo-metasone dipropionate	Inhaled	Generic	MDI	50, 100, 200, 250 µg/puff	Used for asthma prophylaxis from Step 2 onwards (see *Asthma*). Steps 2/3 up to 800 µg/day (children 400 µg/day). Steps 4/5 up to 2000 µg/day (children 800 µg/day).		Hoarseness of voice, oral thrush. Small increased risk of glaucoma, cataract. At higher dosages (> 800 µg/day or > 400 µg/day in children), adrenal suppression and osteoporosis. Monitor growth in children.
			DPI	100, 200, 400 µg/puff			
		Cyclocaps for Cyclohaler	DPI	100, 200, 400 µg/puff			
		AeroBec 50 Autohaler	BAMDI	50 µg/puff	Always use spacer (and face mask for small children) with MDI (except Qvar). Step dosages up or down systematically according to symptoms and lung function (see *Asthma*). Dosages generally divided twice daily, once daily in milder disease		
		AeroBec 100 Autohaler	BAMDI	100 µg/puff			

Inhaled corticosteroids for asthma

Drug	Format	Trade name	Preparation	Strengths	Dosages	Comments	Side effects
Beclo-metasone dipropionate	Inhaled	AeroBec Forte Autohaler	BAMDI	250 µg/puff	Used for asthma prophylaxis from Step 2 onwards (see *Asthma*) Steps 2/3 up to 800 µg/day (children 400 µg/day). Steps 4/5 up to 2000 µg/day (children 800 µg/day).		Hoarseness of voice, oral thrush. Small increased risk of glaucoma, cataract. At higher dosages (> 300 µg/day or > 400 µg/day in children), adrenal suppression and osteoporosis. Monitor growth in children.
		Asmabec Clickhaler	DPI	50, 100, 250 µg/puff			
		Beclazone Easi-Breathe	BAMDI	50, 100, 200, 250 µg/puff			
		Beccdisks for Diskhaler	DPI	100, 200, 400 µg/puff	Always use spacer (and face mask for small children) with MDI (except Qvar). Step dosages up or down systematically according to symptoms and lung function (see *Asthma*). Dosages generally divided twice daily, once daily in milder disease.		
		Becotide 50	MDI	50 µg/puff			
		Becotide 100	MDI	100 µg/puff			
		Becotide 200	MDI	200 µg/puff			
		Beclcforte	MDI	250 µg/puff			
		Qvar 50	MDI	50 µg/puff			
		Qvar 100	MDI	100 µg/puff			
		Qvar 50 Autohaler	BAMDI	50 µg/puff			
		Qvar 100 Autohaler	BAMDI	100 µg/puff			

Inhaled corticosteroids for asthma

Drug	Format	Trade name	Preparation	Strengths	Dosages	Comments	Side effects
Budesonide	Inhaled	Cyclocaps for Cyclohaler	DPI	200, 400 µg/puff	As for beclomethasone (see above)		Hoarseness of voice, oral thrush. Small increased risk of glaucoma, cataract. At higher dosages (> 800 µg/day or > 400 µg/day in children), adrenal suppression and osteoporosis. Monitor growth in children.
		Pulmicort LS	MDI	50 µg/puff			
		Pulmicort	MDI	200 µg/puff			
		Pulmicort Turbohaler	DPI	100, 200, 400 µg/puff			
	Nebulized	Pulmicort	Respule	500, 1000 µg/respule	500–2000 µg twice daily	Not recommended	
Fluticasone propionate	Inhaled	Flixotide Accuhaler	DPI	50, 100, 250, 500 µg/puff	As for beclometasone (see above). Fluticasone is twice as potent as beclometasone or budesonide, so maximum dosages and child dosages should be halved. Accuhaler 250/500 µg, Diskhaler 250/500 µg. Evohaler 125/250 µg per puff preparations are not indicated for children. High topical potency and low bioavailability.		
		Flixotide	MDI	25 µg/puff			
		Flixotide Diskhaler	DPI	50, 100, 250, 500 µg/puff			
		Flixotide Evohaler	MDI	50, 125, 250 µg/puff			
	Nebulized	Flixotide	Nebule	500, 2000 µg nebule	500– 2000 µg twice daily	Not recommended	
Mometasone furoate	Inhaled	Asmanex Twisthaler	DPI	200, 400 µg/puff	Mometasone is more potent than beclometasone and budesonide, but true dosage equivalence is not yet established. High topical potency and particularly low bioavailability. Recommended dosage is 200–400 µg once or twice daily. Not recommended for children.		

Combined preparations of inhaled steroids and long-acting β-agonists for asthma

Drug	Format	Trade name	Preparation	Strengths	Dosages	Comments	Side effects
Budesonide + Formoterol fumarate	Inhaled	Symbicort 100/6 Turbohaler	DPI	Budesonide 80 µg/puff, formoterol 4.5 µg/puff	Adults and children > 6 yr, 1–2 puffs twice daily	Useful for asthma medication at Step 3 and above (see *Asthma*). May aid compliance and reduce prescription charges compared with each drug used separately. MDI devices should be used with a spacer. For mild, well controlled disease, the lowest dosages of Symbicort and Seretide may be used once daily.	See those of separate drugs.
		Symbicort 200/6 Turbohaler	DPI	Budesonide 160 µg/puff, Formoterol 4.5 µg/puff	Adults and children > 12 yr, 1–2 puffs twice daily		
Fluticasone + Salmeterol	Inhaled	Seretide 100 Accuhaler	DPI	Fluticasone 100 µg/puff, Salmeterol 50 µg/puff	Adults and children > 4 yr, 1 puff twice daily		
		Seretide 250 Accuhaler	DPI	Fluticasone 250 µg/puff, Salmeterol 50 µg/puff	Adults and children > 12 yr, 1 puff twice daily		
		Seretide 500 Accuhaler	MDI	Fluticasone 500 µg/puff, Salmeterol 50 µg/puff	Adults and children > 12 yr, 1 puff twice daily		
		Seretide 50 Evohaler	MDI	Fluticasone 50 µg/puff, Salmeterol 25 µg/puff	Adults and children > 12 yr, 2 puffs twice daily		
		Seretide 125 Evohaler	MDI	Fluticasone 125 µg/puff, Salmeterol 25 µg/puff	Adults and children > 12 yr, 2 puffs twice daily		
		Seretide 250 Evohaler	MDI	Fluticasone 250 µg/puff, Salmeterol 25 µg/puff	Adults and children > 12 yr, 2 puffs twice daily		

Drug	Format	Trade name	Preparation	Strengths	Dosages	Comments	Side effects
Leukotriene receptor antagonists for asthma							
Montelukast	Oral	Singulair	Chewable tablet / Tablet	4 mg, 5 mg / 10 mg	10mg once daily (child 2–5yr 4 mg daily; 6–14 yr 5 mg daily)	2nd or 3rd-line "add-on" therapy for asthma at Step 3 or above (see *Asthma*) but not always effective in reducing existing corticosteroid therapy.	Avoid in pregnancy and breast-feeding unless essential. Watch for Churg-Strauss syndrome.
Zafirlukast	Oral	Accolate	Tablet	20 mg	20 mg twice daily (child < 12 yr not recommended)		Avoid in pregnancy and breast-feeding. Contraindicated in hepatic impairment. Watch for Churg-Strauss syndrome.
Cromones for asthma							
Sodium Cromoglicate	Inhaled	Generic Cromogen Easi-Breathe Intal with Syncroner or Fisonair spacer	MDI BAMDI	5 mg/puff 5 mg/puff	5–10 mg 4 times daily and before exercise (adult and child)	4th-line "add-on" therapy for asthma at Step 4 or above (see *Asthma*); not always of benefit; less effective than inhaled corticosteroids when used alone. Nebulized forms are for young children.	Coughing Transient bronchospasm Throat irritation Nedocromil may also cause headache, nausea, vomiting and tastes unpleasant (masked by mint flavouring)
		Intal Spincaps for Spinhaler Insufflator	MDI DPI	5 mg/puff 20 mg/puff	40 mg 4 times daily (adult and child)		
	Nebulized	Generic Intal	Nebulized Nebulized	20 mg/2 ml 20 mg/2 ml	20 mg 4 times daily (adult and child)		
Nedocromil Sodium	Inhaled	Tilade with Syncroner spacer	MDI	2 mg/puff	4 mg 4 times daily (adults and children >6 yr)		

Drug	Format	Trade name	Preparation	Strengths	Dosages	Comments	Side effects
Non-sedating anti-histamines for allergic rhinitis and other allergic diseases							
Acrivastine	Oral	Benadryl Allergy Relief (OTC)	Capsule	8 mg	8 mg 3 times daily (not recommended in children <12 yr. elderly)	Used for allergic rhinitis and conjunctivitis. urticaria and less severe allergic reactions to stings, foods, drugs, latex, etc.	Drowsiness is rare but may occur: advise care with skilled tasks
Cetirizine hydrochloride	Oral	Generic (also OTC)	Tablet	10 mg	10 mg daily (child 2–6 yr 5 mg daily)		Avoid acrivastine, reduce dose of cetirizine, desloratadine, levocetirizine in renal impairment
		Zirtek	Syrup	5 mg/5 ml			
Desloratadine	Oral	Neoclarityn	Tablet	5 mg	5 mg daily (children 6–11yr 2.5 mg daily, 2–5yr 1.25 mg daily)		Manufacturers of cetirizine, desloratadine, fexofenadine, loratadine advise avoidance in pregnancy and breast-feeding
			Syrup	2.5 mg/5 ml			
Fexofenadine	Oral	Telfast 120	Tablet	120 mg	120 mg daily 180 mg daily for urticaria (if <12 yr not recommended)		
		Telfast 180	Tablet	180 mg			
Levocetirizine hydrochloride	Oral	Xyzal	Tablet	5 mg	5 mg daily (adults and children > 6 yr)		
Loratadine	Oral	Generic (also OTC)	Tablet	10 mg	10 mg daily (children 2–6 yr 5 mg daily)		
		Clarityn	Syrup	5 mg/5 ml			

Drug	Format	Trade name	Preparation	Strengths	Dosages	Comments	Side effects
Topical nasal anti-histamines for allergic rhinitis							
Azelastine hydrochloride	Topical	Rhinolast (also OTC)	Nasal spray	140 µg/spray	1 spray each nostril twice daily (adults and children > 5 yr)	Suitable for mild disease. Regular treatment preferable.	Local irritation, occasional drowsiness.
Levocabastine	Topical	Livostin (also OTC)	Nasal spray	0.05% solution	2 sprays each nostril twice daily (adults and children > 9 yr)	Relieve nasal symptoms only.	
Topical nasal steroids for allergic rhinitis							
Beclo-metasone dipropionate	Topical	Generic (also OTC)	Nasal spray	50 µg/spray	2 sprays each nostril twice daily (adults and children > 6yr). Reduce if control achieved.	OTC for adults > 18 yr only. Treatment of choice for moderate to severe allergic rhinitis (for seasonal symptoms commence 2–3 wk in advance; for perennial symptoms use continuously). Avoid in untreated infections and soon after surgery.	Systemic side effects may occur at high dosages. Monitor growth in children. Systemic absorption is particularly likely with drops which should be used for short periods to relieve severe symptoms or polyps.
		Beconase	Nasal spray	50 µg/spray			
Budesonide	Topical	Generic (also OTC)	Nasal spray	100 µg/spray	One spray each nostril twice daily (adults and children > 12 yr). Once daily if control achieved.		Local crusting and bleeding may occur initially, rarely nasal septal perforation and glaucoma.
		Rhinocort Aqua	Nasal spray				
Flunisolide	Topical	Syntaris	Nasal spray	25 µg/spray	2 sprays each nostril twice daily (children 5–14 yr 1 spray twice daily)		
Fluticasone propionate	Topical	Flixonase	Nasal spray	50 µg/spray	2 sprays each nostril once daily (children 4–11yr 1 spray once daily)		
		Flixonase nebule	Nasal drops	400 µg/dose	6 drops each nostril once or twice daily for 4–6 wk (not children)		

Drug	Format	Trade name	Preparation	Strengths	Dosages	Comments	Side effects
Topical nasal steroids for allergic rhinitis							
Mometasone Furoate	Topical	Nasonex	Nasal spray	50 µg/spray	2 sprays each nostril once daily reduced to 1 spray once daily if control achieved	OTC for adults > 18 yr only. Treatment of choice for moderate to severe allergic rhinitis (for seasonal symptoms commence 2–3 wk in advance; for perennial symptoms use continuously). Avoid in untreated infections and soon after surgery.	Systemic side effects may occur at high dosages. Monitor growth in children. Systemic absorption is particularly likely with drops which should be used for short periods to relieve severe symptoms or polyps. Local crusting and bleeding may occur initially, rarely nasal septal perforation and glaucoma.
Triamcinolone acetonide	Topical	Nasacort	Nasal spray	55 µg/spray	(children 6–11 yr 1 spray once daily)		
Betamethasone sodium phosphate	Topical	Betnesol	Nasal drops	0.1% solution	2–3 drops each nostril twice daily		
	Topical	Vista-Methasone	Nasal drops	0.1% solution			
Topical nasal cromoglicate for allergic rhinitis							
Sodium cromoglicate	Topical	Rynacrom	Nasal spray	4% spray	1 spray each nostril 4–6 times daily.	Less effective than topical steroids. Must be used frequently and regularly. May be preferred in children to reduce steroid "load".	Local irritation Occasional bronchospasm
	Topical	Vividrin	Nasal spray	2% spray	1 spray each nostril 4–6 times daily		

Drug	Format	Trade name	Preparation	Strengths	Dosages	Comments	Side effects
Topical nasal decongestants							
Ephedrine hydrocholoride	Topical	Generic	Nasal drops	0.5%, 1% solution	1–2 drops up to 4 times daily. Avoid in infants.	For short-term (maximum 7 days) relief of nasal congestion (e.g. when flying)	Prolonged use causes rebound congestion on withdrawal (rhinitis medicamentosa). May cause local irritation, headache.
Xylometazoline hydrochloride	Topical	Generic	Nasal drops / Paediatric nasal drops	0.1% solution / 0.05% solution	2–3 drops up to 3 times daily (> 12 yr only) / 1–2 drops twice daily (not infants)		
Ipratropium bromide	Topical	Rinatec	Nasal Spray	21 µg/spray	2 sprays each nostril 2–3 times daily (not children <12 yr)	Useful adjunctive treatment for watery rhinorrhoea of any cause	Nasal dryness Epistaxis
Topical ocular anti-histamines for allergic conjunctivitis							
Azelastine hydrocholoride	Topical	Optilast	Eye drops	0.05% solution	2 drops each eye twice daily (> 4 yr only)	Probably more effective than cromoglicate in seasonal and perennial allergic conjunctivitis because action more prolonged – use regularly	Mild irritation Bitter taste
Levocabastine hydrochloride	Topical	Livostin (also OTC)	Eye drops	0.05% solution	2 drops each eye twice daily (> 9 yr only) OTC > 12 yr only		Mild irritation Blurred vision Local oedema
Ketotifen fumarate	Topical	Zaditen	Eye drops	250 µg/ml	2 drops each eye twice daily (child >3 yr only)		Stinging, corneal erosion, dry eye with subconjunctival bleeding
Lodoxamide trometamol	Topical	Alomide	Eye drops	0.1% solution	1–2 drops each eye 4 times daily (> 4 yr only)		Mild transient stinging

Drug	Format	Trade name	Preparation	Strengths	Dosages	Comments	Side effects
Topical ocular cromones for allergic conjunctivitis							
Sodium Cromoglicate	Topical	Generic (also OTC)	Eye drops	2% solution	1–2 drops both eyes at least 4 times daily	Must be used regularly and frequently to be effective	Transient mild irritation
Nedocromil sodium	Topical	Rapitil	Eye drops	2% solution	1–2 drops both eyes 2–4 times daily (> 6 yr only)		
Sedating anti-histamines for emergency treatement of anaphylaxis							
Chlor-pheniramine maleate	Oral	Generic (also OTC)	Tablet	4 mg	4 mg up to 6 times daily (children 1–2yr 1 mg twice daily)	Used orally or parenterally for allergic emergencies, usually in conjunction with intramuscular adrenaline. Syrup also used for milder allergic reactions in children. Can be used for allergic rhinitis, urticaria.	Sedating in many patients (increased by alcohol): avoid skilled tasks and driving. Considered safe in pregnancy and breast-feeding.
			solution	2 mg/5 ml			
		Piriton	Tablet	4 mg	2–5 yr 1 mg up to 6 times daily, 6–12 yr 2 mg up to 6 times daily		
			Syrup	2 mg/5 ml			
	Parenteral	Generic	Injection	10 mg/ml	10–20 mg IM or SC 10–20 mg IV (children 1–5 yr 2.5–5 mg, 6–12 yr 5–10 mg)		

Adrenaline auto-injector pens for anaphylaxis

Drug	Format	Trade name	Preparation	Strengths	Dosages	Comments	Side effects
Adrenaline	Parenteral	Anapen	Intramuscular injection	0.3 mg	For adults and children > 30 kg	For individuals at risk of acute anaphylaxis – administered to anterolateral thigh. Smaller dosages for children < 15kg.	Patients on β-blockers may not respond – consider using salbutamol by infusion or nebulizer instead. Patients on tricyclic anti-depressants more susceptible to arrhythmias – reduce dosage.
		Anapen Junior		0.15 mg	For children 15–30kg		
		Epipen		0.3 mg	For adults and children > 30 kg		
		Epipen Junior		0.15 mg	For children 15–30 kg		

Emollients for eczema: creams, lotions and ointments

Drug	Format	Trade name	Preparation	Strengths	Dosages	Comments	Side effects
	Topical	Aqueous cream BP	Cream		Generics prescribed in multiples of 100 g/100 ml. Others in fixed quantities: Alcoderm (60 g cream, 200 ml lotion); Dermamist (250 ml pressurized aerosol); E45 (50 g, 125 g, 350 g, 500 g cream, 250 ml wash cream, 200 ml, 500 ml lotion); Epaderm (125 g, 500 g ointment); Oilatum (40 g, 150 g cream, 125 g shower gel); Vaseline Dermacare (150 ml cream, 75 ml, 200 ml lotion). Adults: for twice daily application for 1 wk, approximate quantities required are 30 g (face), 50 g (hands). 100 g (scalp), 50 g (hands), 100 g (scalp), 200 g (both arms and legs), 400 g (trunk), 25 g groins and genitalia).	Soothe and hydrate skin in eczema. Should be used frequently. Use creams and ointments as soap substitutes. Use continually even if other therapy, such as topical steroids, prescribed. Use antibacterial additives (see Dermol below) only if widespread or recurrent infection complicates eczema.	Excipients in some preparations rarely cause sensitization and contact dermatitis, in which case avoid.
		Emulsifying ointment BP	Ointment				
		Hydrous ointment BP	Ointment				
		White soft paraffin BP	Ointment				
		Alcoderm	Cream				
			Lotion				
		Cetraben	Cream				
		Dermamist	Lotion spray				

Drug	Format	Trade name	Preparation	Strengths	Dosages	Comments	Side effects
Emollients for eczema: creams, lotions and ointments							
	Topical	Diprobase	Cream		Generics prescribed in multiples of 100 g/100 ml. Others in fixed quantities: Alcoderm (60 g cream, 200 ml lotion); Dermamist (250 ml pressurized aerosol); E45 (50 g, 125 g, 350 g, 500 g cream, 250 ml wash cream, 200 ml, 500 ml lotion); Epaderm (40 g, 150 g, 500 g ointment); Oilatum (40 g, 150 g cream, 125 g shower gel); Vaseline Dermacare (150 ml cream, 75 ml, 200 ml lotion). Adults: for twice daily application for 1 wk. approximate quantities required are 30 g (face), 50 g (hands), 100 g (scalp), 50 g (hands), 100 g (scalp), 200 g (both arms and legs), 400 g (trunk), 25 g (groins and genitalia).	Soothe and hydrate skin in eczema. Should be used frequently. Use creams and ointments as soap substitutes. Use continually even if other therapy, such as topical steroids, prescribed. Use anti-bacterial additives (see Dermol below) only if widespread or recurrent infection complicates eczema.	Excipients in some preparations rarely cause sensitisation and contact dermatitis, in which case avoid.
			Ointment				
		E45	Cream				
			Wash cream				
			Lotion				
		Epaderm	Ointment				
			Cream				
		Oilatum	Cream				
			Shower cream				
		Vaseline Dermacare	Cream				
			Lotion				
		Dermol 500	Lotion			Contains benzalkonium chloride 0.1%, chlorhexidine 0.1%	
		Dermol 200	Shower lotion				

Drug	Format	Trade name	Preparation	Strengths	Dosages	Comments	Side effects
Emollients for eczema: bath additives							
	Topical	Aveeno	Bath oil		30 ml/bath (infants 5 ml)	Use regularly in combination with creams and ointments as soap substitutes. Use antimicrobial additives (below) only if widespread or recurrent infection complicates eczema.	
			Bath additive		1 sachet/bath (infants 0.5 sachet)		
		Balneum Balneum Plus	Bath oil		20 ml/bath (infants 5 ml)		
		Diprobath	Bath additive		25 ml/bath (infants 10 ml)		
		E45	Bath oil		15 ml/bath (children 5–10 ml)		
		Hydromol Emollient	Bath additive		1–3 capfuls/bath (infants 0.5–2)		
		Imuderm	Bath oil		15–30 ml/bath (children 7.5–15 ml)		
Emollients for eczema: bath additives with antimicrobials							
	Topical	Dermol 600	Bath emollient		30 ml/bath (infants 15 ml)	Contains benzalkonium chloride 0.5%	
		Emulsiderm	Bath emulsion		7–30 ml/bath	Contains benzalkonium chloride 0.5%	
		Oilatum Plus	Bath additive		1–2 capfuls/bath (infants > 6 mo 1 ml)	Contains benzalkonium chloride 6%, triclosan 2%	

Topical corticosteroids for eczema: mild potency

Drug	Format	Trade name	Preparation	Strengths	Dosages	Comments	Side effects
Hydro-cortisone	Topical	Generic	Cream Ointment	0.5%, 1% 0.5%, 1%	Apply thinly 1–2 times daily. Adults: for twice daily application for 1 wk, approximate quantities required are 30 g (face and neck), 30 g (both hands), 30 g (both arms), 60 g (both arms), 100 g (both legs), 100 g (trunk), 30 g (groins and genitalia).		Skin atrophy Acreform pustules Peri-oral dermatitis Striae Telangiectasia
		Lanacort (also OTC)	Cream Ointment	1% 1%			
		Hc45 (also OTC)	Cream	1%	Use cream for moist and weeping lesions, ointment for dry and scaly lesions, lotion for large areas and the scalp.		Worsening of existing local infection
		Zenoxone (also OTC)	Cream	1%			Suppression of endogenous cortisol
		Eurax HC (also OTC)	Cream	0.25%			All effects least likely with mild potency drugs. Use these wherever possible for infants and for the face and genitalia.
		Dermacort (also OTC)	Cream	0.1%			
		Dioderm	Cream	1% (equ.)			
		Eurax Hydrocortisone	Cream	0.25%			Contact sensitivity may occur to excipients. If so, use alternative.
		Efcortelan	Cream Ointment	0.5% 0.5%			
		Mildison	Cream	0.1%			

Topical corticosteroids for eczema: mild potency with antimicrobials

Drug	Format	Trade name	Preparation	Strengths	Dosages	Comments	Side effects
Hydro-cortisone	Topical	Canesten HC	Cream	1%	As above. Use only for short periods, preferably for proven superadded bacterial or fungal infection in eczema. Oral antibiotics may be preferable for Staphylococcal infection. Antifungals maybe used for seborrhoeic eczema of the face and scalp (*Malassezia* infection). Also use antifungal shampoos.	Clotrimazole 1%	As above. In addition, contact sensitivity to antimicrobials may occur with prolonged use.
		Daktacort	Cream	1%		Miconazole 2%	
			Ointment	1%			
		Econacort	Cream	1%		Econazole 1%	
		Fucidin H	Cream	1%		Fusidic acid 2%	
			Ointment	1%			
		Gregoderm	Ointment	1%		Neomycin 0.4%, nystatin 10⁵ U/g, polymyxin B 7250U/g	
		Nystaform-HC	Cream	0.5%		Nystatin 10⁵ U/g, chlorhexidine 1%	
		Terra-cortril	Ointment	1%		Oxytetracycline 3%	
			Ointment	1%			
		Terra-cortril Nystatin	Cream	1%		Oxytetracycline 3% nystatin 10⁵ U/g	
		Timodine	Cream	0.5%		Nystatin 10⁵ U/g, benzalkonium chloride 0.2%	
		Vioform -Hydrocortisone	Cream	1%		Clioquinol 3%	
			Ointment	1%			

Drug	Format	Trade name	Preparation	Strengths	Dosages	Comments	Side effects
Topical corticosteroids for eczema: moderate potency							
Hydrocortisone	Topical	Alphaderm	Cream	1%	As above	10% urea increases absorption of steroid	As above. Side effects more likely with higher potency steroids.
		Calmurid HC	Cream	1%	Apply thinly twice daily		
Alclometasone dipropionate	Topical	Modrasone	Cream Ointment	0.05% 0.05%			
Clobetasone butyrate	Topical	Eumovate (cream also OTC > 12 yr)	Cream Ointment	0.05% 0.05%			
		Trimovate	Cream	0.05%		Oxytetracycline 3%	
Desoximetasone	Topical	Stiedex	Cream	0.05%		See comments above regarding the use of additional topical antibacterial and antifungal agents.	
Fludroxycortide	Topical	Haelan	Cream Ointment	0.0125% 0.0125%			
Fluocinolone acetonide	Topical	Synalar 1 in 4 Dilution	Cream Ointment	0.00625% 0.00625%			
Fluocortolone	Topical	Ultralanum Plain	Cream Ointment	0.25% 0.25%			
Betamethasone	Topical	Betnovate-RD	Cream Ointment	0.025% 0.025%			

Topical corticosteroids for eczema: high potency

Drug	Format	Trade name	Preparation	Strengths	Dosages	Comments	Side effects
Hydrocortisone butyrate	Topical	Locoid	Cream Ointment Lotion	0.1% 0.1% 0.1%	As above Apply thinly twice daily	See comments above regarding additional use of topical antibacterial or antifungal agents	As above. Side effects particularly likely. Use only on lichenified eczema, scalp, limbs and trunk. Effect may be increased by occluding with zinc and ichthammol bandage.
Beclometasone dipropionate	Topical	Propaderm	Cream Ointment	0.025% 0.025%			
Betamethasone	Topical	Generic	Cream Ointment	0.1% 0.1%			
		Betacap	Lotion	0.1%			
		Betnovate	Cream Ointment Lotion	0.1% 0.1% 0.1%			
		Bettamousse	Scalp foam	0.1%			
		Diprosone	Cream Ointment Lotion	0.1% 0.1% 0.1%			
		Betnovate -C	Cream Ointment	0.1% 0.1%		Clioquinol 3%	
		Betnovate -N	Cream Ointment	0.1% 0.1%		Neomycin 0.5%	
		FuciBET	Cream	0.1%		Fusidic acid 2%	
		Lotriderm	Cream	0.05%		Clotrimazole 1%	

Drug	Format	Trade name	Preparation	Strengths	Dosages	Comments	Side effects
Topical corticosteroids for eczema: high potency							
Desoximetasone	Topical	Stiedex	Lotion	0.25%			
Fluocinolone acetonide	Topical	Synalar	Cream Gel Ointment	0.025% 0.025% 0.025%			
		Synalar C	Cream Ointment	0.025% 0.025%		Clioquinol 3%	
		Synalar N	Cream Ointment	0.025% 0.025%		Neomycin 0.5%	
Diflucortolone valerate	Topical	Nerisone	Cream Ointment	0.1% 0.1%			
		Nerisone Forte	Cream Ointment	0.3% 0.3%			
Fluocinonide	Topical	Metosyn	Cream Ointment	0.05% 0.05%			
Fluticasone propionate	Topical	Cutivate	Cream Ointment	0.05% 0.005%			
Mometasone furoate	Topical	Elocon	Cream Ointment Lotion	0.1% 0.1% 0.1%			
Triamcinolone acetonide	Topical	Aureocort	Ointment	0.1%		Chlortetracyline 3%	

Drug	Format	Trade name	Preparation	Strengths	Dosages	Comments		Side effects
Topical corticosteroids for eczema: very high potency								
Clobetasol propionate	Topical	Dermovate	Cream Ointment Lotion	0.05% 0.05% 0.05%	As above. Apply thinly twice daily.			Side effects extremely likely. Use for short periods on lichenified eczema, scalp, limbs and trunk and for acute exacerbations.
		Dermovate-NN	Cream Ointment	0.05% 0.05%			Neomycin 0.5%, nystatin 10⁵U/g	
Diflucortolone valerate	Topical	Nerisone Forte	Cream Ointment	0.3% 0.3%				
Halcinonide	Topical	Halciderm Topical	Cream	0.1%				
Topical immunosuppressants for eczema								
Pimecrolimus	Topical	Elidel	Cream	1%	Apply twice daily (not for children < 2yr)	Short-term treatment of eczema. Should be prescribed and managed by specialists (see *Atopic dermatitis*).		Burning Pruritus Skin infections
Tacrolimus	Topical	Protopic	Ointment	0.03%, 0.1%	Adults 0.1% twice daily, then reduce to 0.03% twice daily (children 2–6 yr 0.03% twice daily, then reduce to once daily; not children < 2 yr).			Tacrolimus is contraindicated in pregnancy and breast feeding.

Appendix 2 – Useful websites

World Allergy Organizations
www.worldallergy.org (for health professionals)

www.worldallergy.org/public/allergic_diseases_center/index.shtml (information for the public on allergies referred to different body sites)

Pollen counts and allergens
http://pollenuk.worc.ac.uk (information for doctors and patients on allergy and hayfever, pollen counts in the UK)

www.pollen.com (pollen forecasts for the USA and allergy information)

www.allergen.org (an updated list of major and minor allergens)

www.allergome.org (A very useful list of studies performed on the structure and epidemiology of allergens searched by name, with direct links to published articles)

Professional organizations
These websites contain useful information for health professionals and the general public, including therapy protocols and downloadable information sheets.

www.bsaci.org (British Society for Allergy and Clinical Immunology – contains a list of NHS allergy clinics in the UK)

www.eaaci.org (European Academy of Allergy and Clinical Immunology)

www.aaaai.org (American Academy of Allergy, Asthma and Immunology)

www.nelh.nhs.uk (National Electronic Library for health, providing access to Cochrane databases)

www.brit-thoracic.org.uk (British Thoracic Society, including guidelines on asthma management) www.ersnet.org (European Respiratory Society)

www.lunguk.org (British Lung Foundation)

www.aafa.org (Asthma and Allergy Foundation of America)

www.asthma-carenet.org (Childhood Asthma Research and Education Network)

www.acaai.org (American College of Allergy, Asthma and Immunology)

www.allergy.org.au (Australasian Society for Clinical Immunology and Allergy)

www.aagbi.org (Association of Anaesthetists of Great Britain and Ireland: contains guidelines for documentation and management of anaphylactic reactions during general anaesthesia)

Other organizations providing information for patients and health professionals

www.theallergyreport.org/main.html (Manual of Allergy Diagnosis and Treatment)

www.anaphylaxis.org.uk (website of the Anaphylaxis Campaign, a patient support organization focusing on potentially life threatening allergic reactions)

www.foodallergy.org (Food Allergy and Anaphylaxis network – very useful site for patients with food allergies)

www.lasg.co.uk (Latex Allergy Support Group – support for patients affected by latex allergy)

www.medicalert.org.uk (Registered charity providing a life-saving identification system for patients with serious medical conditions and allergies)

www.asthma.org.uk (National Asthma Campaign – a wealth of information for asthma sufferers and monitoring procedures for health professionals)

www.eczema.org (National Eczema Society – education and training for eczema sufferers) www.allergyfoundation.com (Allergy UK – a patient support organisation with a broad remit encompassing various types of allergy and intolerance)

www.user.globalnet.co.uk (Asthma and Allergy Information and Research: lots of useful information especially for hayfever sufferers)

Information sites provided by pharmaceutical companies

www.actionasthma.co.uk (helpline for asthma patients sponsored by Allen & Hanburys, the respiratory division of GlaxoSmithKline UK)

www.breathingline.co.uk (helpline for asthma patients sponsored by AstraZeneca UK Ltd)

Sites for primary care physicians

www.nrtc.org.uk (National Respiratory Training Centre: training in diagnosis and management of allergic diseases for primary care physicians and practice nurses)

www.gpiag.org (General Practice Airways Group: forum for management of asthma and other respiratory diseases in primary care)

Unproven diagnostic and management techniques

www.quackwatch.com (a regularly updated site providing unbiased evaluation of unproven techniques in the diagnosis and management of allergic and other diseases)

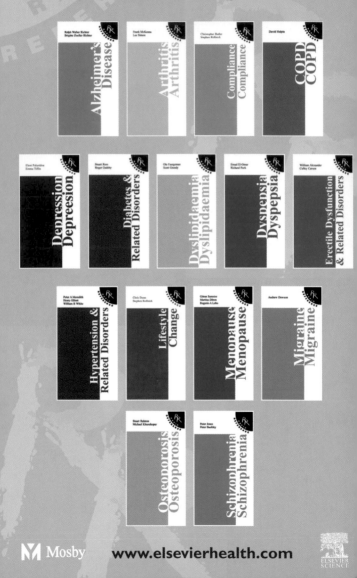

Rapid Reference

A major new series of pocketbooks

Mosby   www.elsevierhealth.com   ELSEVIER SCIENCE

Index

Note:, This index is in letter-by-letter order whereby spaces and hyphens in main entries are excluded from the alphabetization process. Page numbers followed by 'f' indicate figures; page numbers followed by 't' indicate tables.